PREGNANCY AND INFANTS: MEDICAL, PSYCHOLOGICAL AND
SOCIAL ISSUES SERIES

NONMARITAL CHILDBEARING:
TRENDS, REASONS AND POLICY

PREGNANCY AND INFANTS: MEDICAL, PSYCHOLOGICAL AND SOCIAL ISSUES SERIES

Focus on Milk and Infants
Viroj Wiwanitkit
2009. ISBN: 978-1-60741-106-2

Infectious Pregnancy Complications
Richard N. Canfield (Editor)
2009. ISBN: 978-1-60471-038-6

Drugs During Pregnancy
Bengt Källén
2009. ISBN: 978-1-60876-154-8

Breastfeeding: Methods, Benefits to the Infant and Mother, and Difficulties
Wilma G. Nueland (Editor)
2010. ISBN: 978-1-60741-933-4

Human Placenta: Structure and Development, Circulation and Functions
Eirik Berven and Andras Freberg (Editors)
2010. ISBN: 978-1-60876-457-0

Handbook of Prenatal Diagnosis: Methods, Issues and Health Impacts
Elian Pereira and Juliano Soria (Editors)
2010. ISBN: 978-1-60741-254-0

Nonmarital Childbearing: Trends, Reasons and Policy
Gilberto de la Rayes (Editor)
2010. ISBN: 978-1-60741-756-9

PREGNANCY AND INFANTS: MEDICAL, PSYCHOLOGICAL AND
SOCIAL ISSUES SERIES

NONMARITAL CHILDBEARING: TRENDS, REASONS AND POLICY

GILBERTO DE LA RAYES
EDITOR

Nova Science Publishers, Inc.
New York

LIBRARY OF CONGRESS CATALOGING-IN-PUBLICATION DATA
Available upon request

ISBN: 978-1-60741-756-9

Published by Nova Science Publishers, Inc. ✦ New York

CONTENTS

Preface   vii

Chapter 1   Nonmarital Childbearing: Trends, Reasons, and Public
                  Policy Interventions   1
                  Carmen Solomon-Fears

Chapter 2   Reducing Teen Pregnancy: Adolescent Family Life and
                  Abstinence Education Programs   67
                  Carmen Solomon-Fears

Chapter 3   Title X (Public Health Service Act) Family Planning
                  Program   77
                  Angela Napili

Chapter 4   Births: Preliminary Data for 2007   97
                  Brady E. Hamilton, Joyce A. Martin and Stephanie J.
                  Ventura

Index   141

PREFACE

This book explores the significant increase in nonmarital births in the United States, the possible reasons behind the change, and things that can be done to control it. In 2006, a record 38.5% of all United States births were nonmarital births. Many of these children grow up in mother-only families. Although most children who grow up in mother-only families or step-parent families become well-adjusted, productive adults, the bulk of empirical research indicates that children who grow up with only one biological parent in the home are more likely to be financially worse off and have worse socioeconomic outcomes (even after income differences are taken into account) compared to children who grow up with both biological parents in the home. This book analyzes the trends in nonmarital childbearing, discusses some of the characteristics of unwed mothers, addresses some issues involving the fathers of children born outside of marriage, covers many of the reasons for nonmarital childbearing, examines the impact of nonmarital births on families and on the nation, and presents the public policy interventions that have been used to prevent nonmarital births or ameliorate some of the negative financial consequences that are sometimes associated with nonmarital childbearing. This is an edited, excerpted and augmented edition of a NVSR publication.

Chapter 1 - In 2006, a record 38.5% of all United States births were nonmarital births. Many of these children grow up in mother-only families. Although most children who grow up in mother-only families or step-parent families become well-adjusted, productive adults, the bulk of empirical research indicates that children who grow up with only one biological parent in the home are more likely to be financially worse off and have worse socioeconomic outcomes (even after income differences are taken into account) compared to children who grow up with both biological parents in the home.

In recognition of the potential long-term economic and social consequences associated with nonmarital births, the federal government's strategy with regard to nonmarital childbearing has been varied. The federal government recognizes that an effective approach for teenagers may be inappropriate for older women. Federal policy toward teens has primarily focused on pregnancy prevention programs, whereas federal policy toward older women has focused on healthy marriage programs. Federal income support programs are available to mothers of all age groups.

In the U.S., nonmarital births are widespread, touching families of varying income class, race, ethnicity, and geographic area. Many analysts attribute this to changed attitudes about fertility and marriage. They find that many adult women and teenage girls no longer feel obliged to marry before, or as a consequence of, having children. With respect to men, it appears that one result of the so-called sexual revolution is that many men now believe that women can and should control their fertility via contraception or abortion and have become less willing to marry the women they impregnate.

Factors that are associated with the unprecedented level of nonmarital childbearing include an increase in the median age of first marriage (i.e., marriage postponement), decreased childbearing of married couples, increased marital dissolution, an increase in the number of cohabiting couples, increased sexual activity outside of marriage, participation in risky behaviors that often lead to sex, improper use of contraceptive methods, and lack of marriageable partners.

This report analyzes the trends in nonmarital childbearing, discusses some of the characteristics of unwed mothers, addresses some issues involving the fathers of children born outside of marriage, covers many of the reasons for nonmarital childbearing, examines the impact of nonmarital births on families and on the nation, and presents the public policy interventions that have been used to prevent nonmarital births or ameliorate some of the negative financial consequences that are sometimes associated with nonmarital childbearing.

Chapter 2 - In 2007, 48% of students in grades 9-12 reported that they had experienced sexual intercourse; about 20% of female teens who have had sexual intercourse become pregnant each year. In recognition of the often negative, long-term consequences associated with teenage pregnancy, Congress has provided funding for the prevention of teenage and out-of-wedlock pregnancies. This report discusses three programs that exclusively attempt to reduce teenage pregnancy. The Adolescent Family Life (AFL) demonstration program was enacted in 1981 as Title XX of the Public Health Service Act, and the Abstinence Education program was enacted in 1996 as part of the welfare reform legislation. Also, since FY2001, additional funding for community-based abstinence education programs has been included in annual Department of Health and Human Services (HHS) appropriations. This report will be updated periodically.

Chapter 3 - The federal government provides grants for voluntary family planning services through the Family Planning Program, Title X of the Public Health Service Act, codified at 42 U.S.C. § 300 to § 300a-6. The program, enacted in 1970, is the only domestic federal program devoted solely to family planning and related preventive health services. Title X is administered through the Office of Population Affairs (OPA) under the Office of Public Health and Science in the Department of Health and Human Services (DHHS). It receives its funding through appropriations for the Health Resources and Services Administration (HRSA) in DHHS.

Although the authorization for Title X ended with FY1985, funding for the program has continued to be provided through appropriations bills for the Departments of Labor, Health and Human Services, and Education, and Related Agencies (Labor-HHS-Education). The Title X program received $300 million for FY2008, 6% more than the FY2007 level of $283.1 million.

On September 30, 2008, President Bush signed P.L. 110-329, the Consolidated Security, Disaster Assistance, and Continuing Appropriations Act, 2009. P.L. 110-329 provides temporary FY2009 funding, at the FY2008 funding level, through March 6, 2009.

The law (42 U.S.C. § 300a-6) prohibits the use of Title X funds in programs where abortion is a method of family planning. According to OPA, family planning projects that receive Title X funds are closely monitored to ensure that federal funds are used appropriately and that funds are not used for prohibited activities such as abortion. The prohibition on abortion does not apply to all the activities of a Title X grantee, but only to activities that are part of the Title X project. A grantee's abortion activities must be "separate and distinct" from the Title X project activities.

Several bills addressing Title X have been introduced in the 111th Congress. The Prevention First Act (S. 21/H.R. 463) would authorize Title X appropriations of $700 million for FY2010 and "such sums as may be necessary for each subsequent fiscal year." Other introduced bills include H.R. 221, which would require assurances that family planning projects will provide pamphlets with adoption centers' contact information, and S. 85, which would prohibit Title X grants to abortion-performing entities.

In the December 19, 2008 *Federal Register,* DHHS published a rule that is intended to increase awareness of existing statutes that "protect the rights of health care entities/entities, both individuals and institutions, to refuse to perform health care services and research services to which they may object for religious, moral, ethical, or other reasons." Some critics have argued that the rule could limit patients' access to contraception, and that it conflicts with the Title X requirement that grantees provide pregnant women, upon request, nondirective counseling and referrals on several options including abortion.

Chapter 4 – Objectives: This report presents preliminary data for 2007 on births in the United States. U.S. data on births are shown by age, live-birth order, race, and Hispanic origin of mother. Data on marital status, cesarean delivery, preterm births, and low birthweight are also presented.

Methods: Data in this report are based on 98.7 percent of births for 2007. The records are weighted to independent control counts of all births received in state vital statistics offices in 2007. Comparisons are made with 2006 data.

Results: The preliminary estimate of births in 2007 rose 1 percent to 4,317,119, the highest number of births ever registered for the United States. The general fertility rate increased by 1 percent in 2007, to 69.5 births per 1,000 women aged 15–44 years, the highest level since 1990. Increases occurred within all race and Hispanic origin groups and for nearly all age groups. The birth rate for U.S. teenagers 15–19 years rose again in 2007 by about 1 percent, to 42.5 births per 1,000. The birth rate for teenagers 15–17 and 18–19 years each increased by 1 percent in 2007, to 22.2 and 73.9 per 1,000, respectively. The rate for the youngest group, 10–14 years, was unchanged. Birth rates also increased for women in their twenties, thirties, and early forties between 2006 and 2007. The 2007 total fertility rate increased to 2,122.5 births per 1,000 women. All measures of childbearing by unmarried women rose to historic levels in 2007, with the number of births, birth rate, and proportion of births to unmarried women increasing 3 to 5 percent. The cesarean delivery rate rose 2 percent in 2007, to 31.8 percent, marking the 11th consecutive year of increase and another record high for the United States. The rate of preterm births (infants delivered at less than 37 weeks of gestation) decreased 1 percent in 2007, to 12.7 percent, with the decline predominately among infants born late preterm (at 34–36 weeks). The rate of low birthweight (less than 2,500 grams) also declined slightly in 2007, to 8.2 percent.

In: Nonmarital Childbearing: Trends,...   ISBN: 978-1-60741-756-9
Editor: Gilberto de la Rayes   © 2010 Nova Science Publishers, Inc.

Chapter 1

NONMARITAL CHILDBEARING: TRENDS, REASONS, AND PUBLIC POLICY INTERVENTIONS*

Carmen Solomon-Fears
Specialist in Social Policy
Domestic Social Policy Division

SUMMARY

In 2006, a record 38.5% of all United States births were nonmarital births. Many of these children grow up in mother-only families. Although most children who grow up in mother-only families or step-parent families become well-adjusted, productive adults, the bulk of empirical research indicates that children who grow up with only one biological parent in the home are more likely to be financially worse off and have worse socioeconomic outcomes (even after income differences are taken into account) compared to children who grow up with both biological parents in the home.

In recognition of the potential long-term economic and social consequences associated with nonmarital births, the federal government's

---

* This is an edited, reformatted and augmented version of a CRS Report for Congress publication dated November 2008.

strategy with regard to nonmarital childbearing has been varied. The federal government recognizes that an effective approach for teenagers may be inappropriate for older women. Federal policy toward teens has primarily focused on pregnancy prevention programs, whereas federal policy toward older women has focused on healthy marriage programs. Federal income support programs are available to mothers of all age groups.

In the U.S., nonmarital births are widespread, touching families of varying income class, race, ethnicity, and geographic area. Many analysts attribute this to changed attitudes about fertility and marriage. They find that many adult women and teenage girls no longer feel obliged to marry before, or as a consequence of, having children. With respect to men, it appears that one result of the so-called sexual revolution is that many men now believe that women can and should control their fertility via contraception or abortion and have become less willing to marry the women they impregnate.

Factors that are associated with the unprecedented level of nonmarital childbearing include an increase in the median age of first marriage (i.e., marriage postponement), decreased childbearing of married couples, increased marital dissolution, an increase in the number of cohabiting couples, increased sexual activity outside of marriage, participation in risky behaviors that often lead to sex, improper use of contraceptive methods, and lack of marriageable partners.

This report analyzes the trends in nonmarital childbearing, discusses some of the characteristics of unwed mothers, addresses some issues involving the fathers of children born outside of marriage, covers many of the reasons for nonmarital childbearing, examines the impact of nonmarital births on families and on the nation, and presents the public policy interventions that have been used to prevent nonmarital births or ameliorate some of the negative financial consequences that are sometimes associated with nonmarital childbearing. This report will not be updated.

INTRODUCTION

In the United States, being born to an unmarried mother is more likely to lead to less favorable outcomes than is being born to a married mother. In the U.S., births to unmarried women (i.e., nonmarital births) are widespread, touching families of varying income class, race, ethnicity, and geographic area. Many analysts attribute this to changed attitudes about fertility and marriage. They find that many adult women and teenage girls no longer feel obliged to marry before, or as a consequence of, having children. During the 66-year period from 1940 to 2006, the percentage of births to unmarried women increased by a multiple of nine, from 3.8% in 1940 to 38.5% in 2006. This represented about 1.6 million children in 2006.

"Nonmarital births" can be first births, second births, or higher-order births; they can precede a marriage or occur to a woman who has never married. "Nonmarital births" can occur to divorced or widowed women. Moreover, a woman with several children may have had one or more births within marriage and one or more births outside of marriage.[1] Many of the children born outside of marriage are raised by a single parent (who may or may not have a "significant other").[2]

Parents and family life are the foundation that influences a child's well-being throughout the child's development and into adulthood. The family also is the economic unit that obtains and manages the resources that meet a child's basic needs while also playing an instrumental role in stimulating the child's cognitive, social, and emotional development. Children born outside of marriage often are raised solely by their mothers, but sometimes live in other types of family situations. Some are raised solely by their fathers, some are raised by both biological parents who are not married to each other (i.e., cohabiting). Others may be raised by a mother who is living with a male partner. Still others may be living with a mother who is divorced from someone other than their father. Additionally, some may be living with a mother whose husband died (i.e., the mother is a widow but the child was not fathered by the deceased husband).

Although most children who grow up in mother-only families, father-only families, step-parent families, or families in which the mother is cohabiting with a male partner become well-adjusted, productive adults, a large body of research indicates that children who grow up with only one biological parent in the home are more likely to be financially worse off and have worse socioeconomic outcomes (even after income differences are taken into account) compared to children who grow up with both biological parents in the home.[3] To emphasize, this research indicates that all family situations in which both biological parents are not living together (regardless of whether the mother is divorced, separated, widowed, or was never married) are more likely to result in less favorable outcomes for children than a family situation in which the child is living in a household with both biological parents. It is also noteworthy that some researchers conclude that even among children living with both biological parents, living with married parents generally results in better outcomes for children than living with cohabiting parents mainly because marriage is a more stable and longer lasting situation than cohabitation.[4]

The federal concern about nonmarital childbearing centers on its costs via claims on public assistance. These federal costs primarily reflect the fact that many of these "nonmarital children" are raised in single-parent families that are financially disadvantaged. Federal concern also arises because of the aforementioned research indicating that children living in single-parent families are more likely to face negative outcomes (financially, socially, and emotionally) than children who grow up with both of their biological parents in the home. As mentioned earlier, many children born outside of marriage are raised in single-parent families.[5]

This report analyzes the trends in nonmarital childbearing in the U.S., discusses some of the characteristics of unwed mothers, addresses some issues involving the fathers of children born outside of marriage, covers many of the reasons for nonmarital childbearing, examines the impact of nonmarital births on families and on the nation, and presents the public policy interventions that have been used to prevent nonmarital births or alleviate some of the problems that are associated with nonmarital childbearing. This report concludes with commentary on public policy interventions — healthy marriage programs, responsible fatherhood programs, and teen pregnancy prevention strategies — that may receive renewed attention and debate in the 111th Congress.

KEY FINDINGS

Nonmarital childbearing sometimes results in negative outcomes for children mainly because children born outside of marriage are generally not raised by both of their biological parents but rather by single mothers. (Children living in a household maintained by a never-married mother are among the poorest population groups in the U.S.) Even in cases in which cohabiting parents start off raising their children together, it is often of short duration. This section presents some of the major findings of the report.

- After stabilizing in the 1990s, nonmarital births are again increasing. In 2006, 38.5% of all births were nonmarital births. This surpasses the percentage in 1960 that prompted some policymakers to claim that the black family was disintegrating because a large share of nonmarital births were to black women. In 2006, 70.7% of African American births were nonmarital births compared with 64.6% of American Indian births, 49.9% of Hispanic births, 26.6% of white births, and 16.3% of Asian births.[6]

- Nonmarital births can be first births, second births, or higher-order births; they can precede a marriage or occur to a woman who has never married. Nonmarital births can occur to divorced or widowed women. Moreover, a woman with several children may have had one or more births within marriage and one or more births outside of marriage.[7]

- After declining for 14 straight years, *all* teen births increased in 2006. Contrary to public perception, women in their early twenties, not teens, have the highest percentage of births outside of marriage. In 2005, women ages 20 through 24 accounted for 38% of the 1.5 million nonmarital births. The comparable statistic for females under age 20[8] was 23%. However, many women who have nonmarital births in their twenties were also teen moms.[9]

- Births to teenagers are an important component of nonmarital births because more than 80% of births to teenagers are nonmarital births.

- Although women have been postponing marriage, women of all ages do not view marriage as a requirement for sexual activity.[10] With the longer time span between the onset of sexual activity and marriage, the trend of high numbers of nonmarital births may/could continue.

- Although nonmarital births are increasing, many more children than in previous decades live with both biological parents in cohabiting situations for some period of time.

- According to analysts, marriage is considered a better option for children than cohabitation because marriage is more stable (i.e., lasts longer) than cohabiting situations.

- Growing up in a single-parent family is one of many factors that put children at risk of less favorable outcomes. The economic, social, psychological, and emotional costs associated with children with absent noncustodial parents are significant. Nevertheless, most children who grow up in single-parent families become productive adults. Children living in a single-parent home are more likely to do poorly in school, have emotional and behavioral problems, become teenage parents, and have poverty-level income (as children and adults) compared to children living with married biological parents.[11] In 2007, 67.8% of the 73.7 million U.S. children (under age 18) lived with both of their married parents, 2.9% lived with both parents who were not married, 17.9% lived with their mother, and 2.6% lived with their father.

- The advent of multiple relationships that produce children adds complexity to the problem. These relationships, often referred to as multiple partner fertility (i.e., when mothers and fathers have had children with more than one partner), generally complicate the family situation of children.
- Compared to women without nonmarital children, women with children who were born outside of marriage are less like to marry;[12] if they do marry, their spouses are more likely to be economically disadvantaged.[13]
- Demographically, without nonmarital births, the U.S. would be far below population replacement levels. Having the birth rate reach the replacement rate is generally considered desirable by demographers and sociologists because it means a country is producing enough young people to replace and support aging workers without population growth being so high that it taxes national resources.
- Nonmarital births are expected to increase over time because of a projected population shift toward more minorities. The Census Bureau projects that by 2050, 54% of the U.S. population will consist of minority groups (i.e., Hispanics, blacks, Indians, and Asians). Minorities, now roughly one-third of the U.S. population, are expected to become the majority in 2042, with the nation projected to be 54% minority in 2050. By 2023, minorities will represent more than half of all children. The Hispanic population is projected to nearly triple, and its share of the nation's total population is projected to double, from 15% to 30%. Thus, nearly one in three U.S. residents will be Hispanic.[14] In 2005, 48% of Hispanic births were nonmarital births.

TRENDS IN NONMARITAL BIRTHS: 1940-2006

In this report, births to unmarried women are termed nonmarital births. Data on nonmarital births[15] are usually expressed by three measures: the number of nonmarital births, the percent of births that are nonmarital, and the rate of nonmarital births per 1,000 unmarried women.

The number of nonmarital births provides the absolute count of babies who are born to women (including adolescents), who are not married. The percent of all births that are nonmarital[16] is the number of all nonmarital births divided by all births (both nonmarital births and marital births). The nonmarital birth rate is defined as the number of nonmarital births per 1,000 unmarried women.

During the 66-year period from 1940 through 2006, there was a 17-fold increase in the number of babies born to unmarried women living in the United States. The number of babies born to unmarried women increased from 89,500 in 1940 to 1,641,700 in 2006. In 2006, 38.5% of all U.S. births were to unmarried women, up from 3.8% in 1940 — a nine-fold increase.

Numbers, Percentages, and Rates

The number of nonmarital births reached a record high in 2006 with 1,641,700 births to unmarried women. As mentioned above, the number of births to unmarried women has generally increased over the years, with some downward fluctuations.

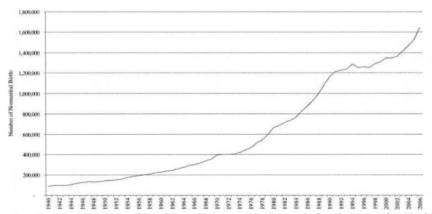

Source: U.S. Department of Health and Human Services, National Center for Health Statistics, "Nonmarital Childbearing in the United States, 1940-99," *National Vital Statistics Reports*, vol. 48, no. 16 (October 18, 2000). See also *National Vital Statistics Reports*, vol. 56, no. 6 (December 5, 2007).

Figure 1. Number of Births to Unmarried Women, 1940-2006

As shown in **Figure 1**, nonmarital births rose 17-fold from 1940-2006. (Also see the data table in **Appendix A**.) The average annual increase in nonmarital births has slowed substantially from earlier decades. The average annual increase in nonmarital births was 4.9% from 1940-1949; 5.6% from 1950-1959; 6.1% from 1960-1969; 5.0% from 1970-1979; 6.4% from 1980-1989; 1.2% from 1990-1999 (and 3.6% for the seven years from 2000-2006). The 1990s showed a marked slowing of nonmarital births, dropping from an average increase of 6.4% a year in the 1980s to an average of 1.2% a year in the 1990s. During the first six years of the 2000 to 2010 period, the average annual increase in nonmarital births increased to 3.6%.

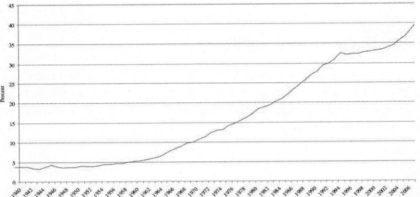

Source: U.S. Department of Health and Human Services, National Center for Health Statistics, "Nonmarital Childbearing in the United States, 1940-99," *National Vital Statistics Reports*, vol. 48, no. 16 (October 18, 2000). See also *National Vital Statistics Reports*, vol. 56, no. 6 (December 5, 2007).

Figure 2. Percentage of Births to Unmarried Women, 1940-2006

The percent of births to unmarried women increased substantially during the period from 1940-2006 (see **Figure 2** and the Appendix table). (However, from 1994-2000, there was almost no change in this measure.) In 1940, 3.8% of all U.S. births were to unmarried women. By 2006, a record 38.5% of all U.S. births were to unmarried women.

The nonmarital birth rate provides a measure of the likelihood that an unmarried woman will give birth in a given year. The birth rate for unmarried women increased dramatically during the 1940-2006 period, with many upward and downward fluctuations. (However, during the years 1995-2002, the nonmarital birth rate remained virtually unchanged.[17]) The nonmarital birth rate increased from 7.1 births per 1,000 unmarried women ages 15 through 44 in 1940 to a record high of 50.6 births per 1,000 women ages 15 through 44 in 2006 (a six-fold increase). (See **Figure 3** and the **Appendix, Table A-1**.)

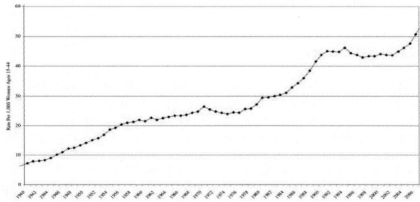

Source: U.S. Department of Health and Human Services, National Center for Health Statistics, "Nonmarital Childbearing in the United States, 1940-99," *National Vital Statistics Reports*, vol. 48, no. 16 (October 18, 2000). See also *National Vital Statistics Reports*, vol. 56, no. 6 (December 5, 2007).

Figure 3. Rate of Births to Unmarried Women, 1940-2006

CHARACTERISTICS OF UNWED MOTHERS

This section discusses some of the characteristics of unmarried mothers. It includes some of the demographic characteristics like race, ethnicity, and age as well as other features like whether the unwed mother has additional children, her income status, whether or not she marries, and whether or not she is in a cohabiting relationship. Some of the highlights include the following:

- black women are more likely to have children outside of marriage than other racial or ethnic groups;
- it is not teenagers but rather women in their early twenties who have the highest percentage of births outside of marriage;
- single motherhood is more common among women with less education than among well-educated women;
- a substantial share of nonmarital births (44%) were to women who had already given birth to one or more children;

- a significant number of unwed mothers are in cohabiting relationships; and
- women who have a nonmarital birth are less likely than other women to eventually marry.

Race and Ethnicity

The rate at which unmarried women have children varies dramatically by race and ethnicity. As mentioned earlier, in 2005, the nonmarital birth rate for all U.S. women was 47.5 births per 1,000 unmarried women.[18] In 2005, Hispanic women had the highest nonmarital birth rate at 100.3 births per 1,000 unmarried women. The nonmarital birth rate in 2005 was 67.8 for black women, 30.1 for non-Hispanic white women, and 24.9 for Asian or Pacific Islander women. Although Hispanic women had the highest nonmarital birth rate, a greater share (percentage) of black women had nonmarital births.

In 2005, 36.9% of all U.S. births were to unmarried women.[19] In 2005, 69.9% of births to black women were nonmarital births. The percentage of nonmarital births for American Indians or Alaska Natives was 63.5%. The nonmarital birth percentage was 48.0% for Hispanic women, 25.3% for non-Hispanic white women, and 16.2% for Asian or Pacific Islander women.[20] (See **Table 1**.)

The greatest share of children born to unmarried women are white; however, minority children, particularly black children and Hispanic children, are overrepresented. Of the 1.5 million children who were born outside of marriage in 2005, 38% were white (whites constituted 80% of the U.S. population), 27% were black (blacks constituted 13% of the population), 2% were American Indian/Alaskan Native (American Indians or Alaskan Natives constituted 1% of the population), 2% were Asian or Pacific Islander (Asians or Pacific Islanders constituted 4% of the population), and 32% were Hispanic (Hispanics constituted 14% of the population).

In 2005, the percentage of nonmarital births to black women (nearly 70%) was more than three times the 22% level of the early 1960s that so alarmed Daniel Patrick Moynihan, then President Johnson's Assistant Secretary of Labor. Moynihan addressed the issue in a report called "The Negro Family: The Case for National Action."[21] One theory that attempts to explain the disproportionate share of nonmarital births to black women hypothesizes that the universe of males (ages 15 and above) who are unmarried is disproportionately lower for blacks. For example, in 2005, there were 74 black unmarried males for every 100 unmarried black females; 87 white non-Hispanic unmarried males for every 100 unmarried white non-Hispanic females; 98 Asian unmarried males for every 100 Asian unmarried females; and 113 Hispanic unmarried males for every 100 Hispanic unmarried females.[22] Supporters of this theory argue that if the universe of possible marriage partners is reduced to desirable marriage partners (e.g., heterosexual men, men with steady jobs, men without a criminal record, and men with a similar educational background), the black "male shortage" is drastically increased.[23]

Age

Teen marriage and birth patterns have shifted from a general trend of marrying before pregnancy, to marrying as a result of pregnancy, to becoming pregnant and not marrying.[24] Early nonmarital childbearing remains an important issue, especially in the U.S., because young first-time mothers are more likely to have their births outside of marriage than within marriage, and because women who have a nonmarital first birth are increasingly likely to have all subsequent births outside of marriage, although often in cohabiting unions.[25]

The proportion of births to unmarried women (i.e., nonmarital births) who are teenagers also has decreased over the last half-century. In 1950, 42% of the 141,600 nonmarital births were to females under age twenty. In 1970, 50% of the 398,700 nonmarital births were to females under age twenty. In 1990, 31% of the nearly 1.2 million (1,165,384) nonmarital births were to females under age twenty. In 2005, 23% of the 1.5 million (1,527,034) nonmarital births in the U.S. were to teenagers.

In contrast, the percentage of *all* teen births that are nonmarital has increased dramatically. In other words, in recent years, most teenagers who give birth are not married. For example, only 13% of the 419,535 babies born to teens (ages 15 to 19) in 1950 were born to females who were not married. Whereas, in 2005, 83% of the 414,593 babies born to teens (ages 15 to 19) were born to unwed teens. There are two reasons for this phenomenon. The first is that marriage in the teen years, which was not uncommon in the 1950s, has become quite rare. (As mentioned earlier, the typical age of first marriage in the U.S. has risen to 25.5 for women and 27.5 for men.) The second is that this general trend of marriage postponement has extended to pregnant teens as well: In contrast to the days of the "shotgun marriage," very few teens who become pregnant nowadays marry before their baby is born.[26]

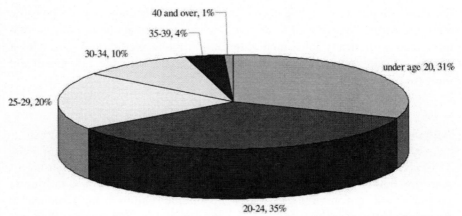

Source: U.S. Department of Health and Human Services, National Center for Health Statistics, "Nonmarital Childbearing in the United States, 1940-99," *National Vital Statistics Reports*, vol. 48, no. 16 (October 18, 2000).

Figure 4. Percentage Distribution of Nonmarital Births, by Age of Mother, 1990

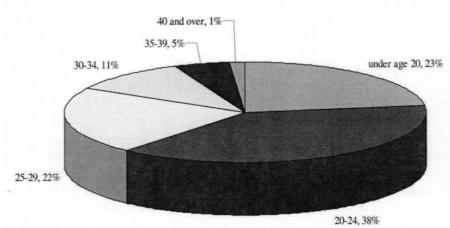

Source: U.S. Department of Health and Human Services, National Center for Health Statistics, "Births: Final Data for 2005," *National Vital Statistics Reports*, vol. 56, no. 6 (December 5, 2007).

Figure 5. Percentage Distribution of Nonmarital Births, by Age of Mother, 2005

Contrary to public perception, it is not teenagers but rather women in their early twenties who have the highest percentage of births outside of marriage. In 1990, 31% of the 1,165,384 nonmarital births in the U.S. were to teenagers (under age 20), 35% were to women ages 20 through 24, 20% were to women ages 25 through 29, 10% were to women ages 30 through 34, 4% were to women ages 35 through 39, and less than 1% were to women ages 40 and above (see **Figure 4**). In 2005, 23% of the 1,527,034 nonmarital births in the U.S. were to teenagers (under age 20),[27] 38% were to women ages 20 through 24, 22% were to women ages 25 through 29, 11% were to women ages 30 through 34, 5% to women ages 35 through 39, and 1% were to women ages 40 and above.[28] (See **Figure 5**.)

Nonetheless, even though the percentage of all nonmarital births to teens has declined, teen mothers are likely to have subsequent births outside of marriage.[29] In 2006, 19% of all teen births were second or higher-order births. According to some research, 20%-37% of adolescent mothers give birth a second time within 24 months.[30] Thus, some of the women who have a nonmarital birth in their early twenties were teenage mothers as well.

An alternate analysis of the age and nonmarital birth data shows that across all age groups a growing share of women are having nonmarital births. In 1990, 67.1% of births to females under age 20 were nonmarital, as were 36.9% of births to women ages 20 through 24, 18.0% of births to women ages 25 through 29, 13.3% of births to women ages 30 through 34, 13.9% of births to women ages 35 through 39, and 17.0% of births to women ages 40 and over. Whereas in 2005, 83.5% of births to females under age 20 were nonmarital, as were 56.2% of births to women ages 20 to 24, 29.3% of births to women ages 25 to 29, 17.0% of births to women ages 30 to 34, 15.7% of births to women ages 35 to 39, and 18.8% of births to women ages 40 and over. (See **Figure 6**.)

Until recently, a commonly held view was that if childbearing was deferred until a woman reaches her early or late twenties, she would most likely be married. Given that nonmarital birth rates and percentages are at their highest recorded levels and that the number of babies born to teenagers has dramatically decreased in fourteen of the last fifteen years, policymakers are faced with a new paradigm of whether to address births outside of marriage for older women. In these times of scarce resources, it is debatable whether a consensus can be garnered for using public funds to educate women in their mid-twenties and thirties about the negative consequences associated with nonmarital births.[31] Many observers hold the view that older women who have children outside of marriage should have known better, or believe that these women have children for selfish reasons and should live with the consequences, without government assistance or interference.[32] Others argue that the motto "in the best interest of the child" should prevail[33] and that if government aid is necessary and appropriate it should be given.

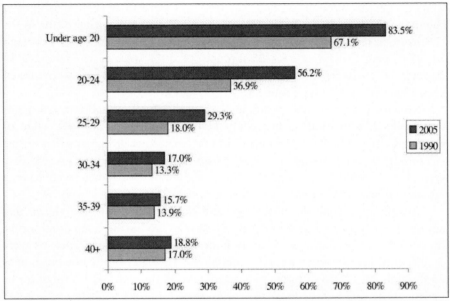

Source: U.S. Department of Health and Human Services, National Center for Health Statistics, "Births: Final Data for 2005," *National Vital Statistics Reports*, vol. 56, no. 6 (December 5, 2007).

Figure 6. Percentage of Births That Are Nonmarital Births, by Age Group, 1990 and 2005

Educational Attainment

Single motherhood has always been more common among women with less education than among well-educated women. But the gap has grown over time. In 1960, 14% of mothers in the bottom quarter of the education distribution were unmarried, as compared to 4.5% of mothers in the top quarter — a difference of 9.5 percentage points. By 2000, the corresponding figures were 43% for the less educated mothers and 7% for the more educated mothers — a gap of 36 percentage points.[34]

Table 1. Percentage of All Births That Were to Unmarried Women, by Race, Ethnicity, and Age, Selected Years 1960-2006

	1960	1970	1980	1985	1990	1995	2000	2003	2004	2005	2006
Total Births	**5.3**	**10.7**	**18.4**	**22.0**	**28.0**	**32.2**	**33.2**	**34.6**	**35.8**	**36.9**	**38.5**
Race/Ethnicity											
White (non-Hispanic)	NA	NA	9.6	12.4	16.9	21.2	22.1	23.6	24.5	25.3	26.6
Black (non-Hispanic)	NA	NA	57.3	62.1	66.7	70.0	68.7	68.5	69.3	69.9	70.7
Hispanic	NA	NA	23.6	29.5	36.7	40.8	42.7	45.0	46.4	48.0	49.9
Asian or Pacific Islander	NA	NA	7.3	9.5	13.3	16.3	14.8	15.0	15.5	16.2	16.3
American Indian or Alaskan Native	NA	NA	39.2	46.8	53.6	57.2	58.4	61.3	62.3	63.5	64.6
Age											
Under 15 years	67.9	80.8	88.7	91.8	91.6	93.5	96.5	97.1	97.4	98.0	98.3
15-19	14.8	29.5	47.6	58.0	67.1	75.2	78.8	81.3	82.4	83.3	84.2
20-24	4.8	8.9	19.4	26.3	36.9	44.7	49.5	53.2	54.8	56.2	57.9
25-29	2.9	4.1	9.0	12.7	18.0	21.5	23.5	26.4	27.8	29.3	31.0
30-34	2.8	4.5	7.5	9.7	13.3	14.7	14.0	15.1	16.1	17.0	18.3
35-39	3.0	5.2	9.4	11.2	13.9	15.7	14.3	14.8	15.2	15.7	16.4
40 years and over	3.1	5.7	12.1	14.0	17.0	18.1	16.8	17.9	18.2	18.8	19.4

Source: Child Trends, Data Bank, Percentage of Births to Unmarried Women. National Center for Health Statistics, National Vital Statistics Reports, vol. 48, no. 16 (October 18, 2000). National Center for Health Statistics, Births: Final Data for 2005, vol. 56, no. 6 (and other selected years). National Vital Statistics Reports, vol. 56, no. 7 (December 5, 2007).
NA = Not available.

Income Status

An examination of never-married mothers shows that in 2007, 41.1% of never-married mother families (with children under age 18) had income below the poverty level. With respect to the various income categories, 23.0% of never-married mother families had income below $10,000, 45.9% had income below $20,000, and 55.1% had income below $25,000; 19.2% had income above $50,000.[35]

Additional Children

Some studies have found that a woman is most likely to have a second birth while in the same type of situation (single, cohabiting, or married) as she was in for the first birth.[36]

The public perception is that nonmarital births are first births. The reality is that in 2005, 44% of the 1.5 million nonmarital births occurred to women who had already given birth to one or more children.[37] In 2007, 46% of mother-only families had more than one child.[38]

Cohabitation

In 2007, 6.4 million family households in the U.S. were classified as unmarried-partner, or cohabiting, households.[39] This represented 8.2% of the 78.4 million U.S. family households.[40] Thirty years earlier, in 1977, only 1.1 million family households consisted of cohabiting couples — this represented 2% of the 56.5 million family households in 1977.[41] A report on trends in cohabitation indicated that cohabitation is now the norm with approximately 54% of all first marriages beginning with a cohabiting relationship. The report estimated that a majority of young men and women of marriageable age today will spend some time in a cohabiting relationship.[42] Cohabiting relationships are generally considered less stable than marriages. According to several sources, cohabiting relationships are fragile and relatively short in duration, with fewer than half lasting five years or more.[43] A 2004 study found that, a year after the birth, 15% of cohabiting couples had married.[44]

The notion that unmarried births equals mother-only families is no longer correct. The decline in the percentage of births to married women has in large measure been in tandem with the increase in births to parents who are living together but who are not married (in cohabiting relationships). According to one study, the proportion of babies of unmarried women born into cohabiting families increased from 29% to 41% from 1980-1984 to 1990-1994, accounting for almost all of the increase in unmarried childbearing over that period.[45] According to Census data, in 2006, approximately 160,000 never-married women (4%) who gave birth within the last 12 months were in a cohabiting relationship.[46]

Some children live with cohabiting couples who are either their own unmarried parents or a biological parent and a live-in partner. Approximately 39% of the 6.4 million unmarried-partner (cohabiting) families in 2007 included biological children (of either the mother or father or both) under the age of 18 (i.e., this amounted to 2.5 million families).[47] This is compared to the 44% of the 58.9 million married-couple families with biological children under age 18 (this amounted to 26.2 million families); and the 60% of the 14.4 million mother-only families with biological children under age 18 (this amounted to 8.6 million families); and the 40% of the 5.1 million father-only families with biological children under age 18 (this amounted to 2.0 million families).[48]

Some analysts contend that the increase in nonmarital childbearing could be seen as less of an issue if viewed through a framework that portrays out-of-wedlock births as babies born to cohabiting couples rather than "single" women. Consistent with the data mentioned earlier, several reports and studies indicate that about 40% of unmarried mothers are cohabiting with the father of their baby, at least at the time of the baby's birth.[49] According to the National Survey of Family Growth, about 9% of annual births to white women were to cohabiting women; among black women, 15% were to cohabiting women; and among Hispanic women, 22% of births occurred to women who were cohabiting.[50]

Others point out that cohabitation is a complex phenomenon that has an array of meanings. Some view it as a precursor to marriage while others view it as an alternative to marriage.[51] According to one study:

> "cohabitation is a continuous rather than a dichotomous variable. At both ends of the continuum, there is substantial agreement across measures about who is (not) cohabiting. In the middle of the continuum, however, there is considerable ambiguity, with as much as 15% of couples reporting part-time cohabitation. How we classify this group will affect estimates of the prevalence of cohabitation, especially among African Americans, and may impact the characteristics and outcomes of cohabitors."[52]

Subsequent Marriage of Mothers

Many women marry after having a child. According to the research, about 40% of unwed mothers marry within five years after giving birth (it is not known whether they marry the father of their child).[53] Yet, women who have a nonmarital birth are less likely than other women ever to marry. A study based on retrospective life histories found that at age 17, girls who had a nonmarital birth were 69% more likely to be never married at age 35 than 17-year old girls who did not have a nonmarital birth (i.e., 24% vs. 14.0%). Women ages 20 to 24 who had a nonmarital birth were more than twice as likely (102%) to not be married at age 35 than women ages 20 to 24 who did not have a nonmarital birth (i.e., 38% vs. 19.0%). The reported implications of these findings is that there probably is a causal relationship between nonmarital childbearing and subsequent marriage.[54]

Another study[55] points out the racial differences associated with the eventual marriage of many women who had a nonmarital birth. The study found that white women were more likely to be married than their minority counterparts. Some 82% of white women, 62% of Hispanics and 59% of blacks who had a nonmarital first birth had married by age 40; the corresponding proportions among those who avoided nonmarital childbearing were 89%, 93% and 76%, respectively.

By some estimates, having a child outside of marriage decreases a woman's chances of marrying by 30% in any given year. Even when they do marry, women who have had a nonmarital birth generally are less likely to stay married. Analysis of data from the 2002 National Survey of Family Growth indicates that women ages 25 to 44 who had their first child before marriage and later got married are half as likely to stay married as women who did not have a nonmarital birth (42% compared to 82%)."[56]

The following section highlights a couple of demographic factors associated with the fathers of children born outside of marriage. It also discusses the importance of establishing paternity for children born outside of marriage.

FATHERS OF CHILDREN BORN OUTSIDE OF MARRIAGE

It has been pointed out that fathers are far too often left out of discussions about nonmarital childbearing. It goes without saying that fathers are an integral factor in nonmarital childbearing. It appears that one result of the so-called sexual revolution was that many men increasingly believed that women could and should control their fertility via contraception and abortion. As a result, many men have become less willing to marry the women they impregnate.[57]

There are myriad reasons why so many children live in homes without their fathers. Some reasons are related to choices people make about fertility, marriage, and cohabitation. But others are the result of unexpected events, such as illness, or incarceration. Some noncustodial fathers are active in the lives of their children, whereas others are either unable or unwilling to be involved in their children's lives. Whatever the reason, a father's absence from the home results in social, psychological, emotional, and financial costs to children and economic costs to the nation. A 2008 report maintains that the federal government spends about $99.8 billion per year in providing financial and other support (via fourteen federal social welfare programs) to father-absent families.[58]

This section of the report discusses the race and ethnicity of fathers to children born outside of marriage, age of fathers, and the importance of establishing paternity for children born outside of marriage. One of the prominent, but perhaps not unexpected, findings related to fathers and nonmarital births is that when older men have sexual relationships with young women it often results in nonmarital births.

Race and Ethnicity

According to the 2002 National Survey of Family Growth, 33% of unmarried Hispanic men and 33% of unmarried non-Hispanic black men have had a biological child, compared with 19% of unmarried non-Hispanic white men. Non-Hispanic black fathers were less likely to be married at the time their first child was born (37%) compared with non-Hispanic white fathers (77%) and Hispanic fathers (52%). A nonmarital first birth was more prevalent among younger fathers, black and Hispanic fathers, and fathers with lower levels of income, and men whose mothers had lower levels of education.[59]

Age

In the United States, it is not unusual for a man to be several years older than his female partner. Some data indicate that the man is three or more years older than the woman in almost four in 10 relationships today. Therefore, it is not unexpected that a similar pattern exists for sexually active teenagers. However, such age differences often have adverse consequences for young women.[60] Several studies have found that the unequal power dynamic that is often present in relationships between teenage girls and older men is more likely to lead to sexual contact not wanted by the female, less frequent use of contraceptives, and a greater incidence of sexually-transmitted diseases (STDs) among the adolescent females.[61]

Further, a significant share of teenagers in relationships with older men have children outside of marriage. According to one study, about 20% of births to unmarried, teenage girls are attributed to men at least five years older than the mother.[62] According to another report, unmarried teenagers younger than 18 were especially likely to become pregnant when involved with an older partner: 69% of those whose partner was six or more years older became pregnant, compared with 23% of those whose partner was three to five years older and 17% of those whose partner was no more than two years older.[63]

Paternity Establishment

Paternity is presumed if a child is conceived within marriage. In other words, the husband is presumed to be the father of a child born to his wife. In cases in which the child is born outside of marriage, paternity can be voluntarily acknowledged or it can be contested. It would be contested in cases in which (1) the mother does not want to establish paternity, thereby forcing the father to take his case to court to assert his rights, (2) the biological father does not want to pay child support and denies paternity to delay establishment of a child support order, or (3) the alleged father has genuine doubt about his paternity. If paternity is contested it is generally resolved through either an administrative process or a judicial proceeding.

A child born outside of marriage has a biological father but not necessarily a legal father. Paternity establishment refers to the legal determination of fatherhood for a child. In 2006, 38.5% of children born in the United States were born to unmarried women, adding approximately 1.6 million new children to the list of children without a legally identified father. Data from the federal Office of Child Support Enforcement (OCSE) indicate that in 2006 the total number of children in the Child Support Enforcement (CSE) caseload[64] who were born outside of marriage amounted to about 10.4 million.[65] Paternity has been established or acknowledged for about 8.9 million (86%) of these children (1.7 million during FY2006), leaving nearly 1.5 million children in the CSE caseload without a legally identified father.[66]

Paternity establishment is not an end in itself, but rather a prerequisite to obtaining ongoing economic support (i.e., child support) from the other (noncustodial) parent.[67] Once paternity is established legally (through a legal proceeding, an administrative process, or voluntary acknowledgment), a child gains legal rights and privileges. Among these may be rights to inheritance, rights to the father's medical and life insurance benefits, and to social security and possibly veterans' benefits. It also may be important for the health of the child for doctors to have knowledge of the father's medical history. The child also may have a chance to develop a relationship with the father and to develop a sense of identity and connection to the "other half" of his or her family.

The public policy interest in paternity establishment is based in part on the dramatic increase in nonmarital births over the last several decades and the economic status of single mothers and their children. The poorest demographic group in the U.S. consists of children in single-parent families. Paternity establishment generally is seen as a means to promote the social goals of (1) providing for the basic financial support of all minor children regardless of the marital status of their parents, (2) ensuring equity in assessing parental liability for the financial support of their children, and (3) promoting responsibility for the consequences of one's actions.[68]

Many observers maintain that the social, psychological, emotional, and financial benefits of having one's father legally identified are irrefutable. They suggest that paternity should be established, regardless of the ability of the father to pay child support. They argue that the role of both parents is critical in building the self-esteem of their children and helping the children become self-sufficient members of the community.

Current literature and studies suggest that in most cases visitation with the noncustodial parent is important to the healthy emotional development of children. Children with regular contact with their noncustodial parent often adjust better than those denied such contact. Moreover, generally it is in the best interest of the child to receive social, psychological, and financial benefits of a relationship with both parents. Visitation (i.e., contact with one's children) is the primary means by which noncustodial parents carry out their parenting duty.[69]

The following section discusses some of demographic factors that have contributed to the increase in nonmarital births as well as some of the reasons, cited by women, for nonmarital childbearing.

REASONS FOR THE INCREASE IN NONMARITAL CHILDBEARING

Declining marriage rates, increased childbearing among unmarried women, increased number of unmarried women in the childbearing ages (i.e., 15-44), and decreased childbearing among married women have contributed to the rising share of children being born to unwed women.

Many social science analysts attribute the increase in nonmarital births to the decades-long decline of "shotgun marriages," rather than to an increased incidence of nonmarital conceptions. They contend thatwhen the social pressure to get married once pregnancy became obvious ended, the likelihood that women would marry between conception and birth decreased substantially.[70] The entry of more and more women into the paid labor force also made childbearing outside of marriage more economically feasible.

Through the 1960s, most Americans believed that parents should stay in an unhappy marriage for the sake of the children. By the 1970s, this view was not as prominent. Divorce and not getting married to the father of a child — which were generally considered to not be in the best interest of the child — were acceptable if it resulted in the happiness of the adult. Thus, many observers and analysts agree that marriage is now more likely to be viewed through a framework of adult fulfillment rather than through a framework of childbearing and childrearing.[71]

Factors that have contributed to an unprecedented level of nonmarital childbearing include an increase in the median age of first marriage (i.e., marriage postponement), delays in childbearing of married couples, increased marital dissolution, an increase in the number of cohabiting couples, increased sexual activity outside of marriage, participation in risky behaviors that often lead to sex, improper use of contraceptive methods,[72] and lack of marriageable partners. This section of the report does not try to verify, refute, or support any of the reasons commonly cited for nonmarital births. Instead, its purpose is to give the reader a better understanding of the nonmarital birth phenomenon by synthesizing and simplifying the large body of research on the subject and presenting the views of analysts and other observers in a way that helps to clarify the complexity of the topic.

Demographic Factors Contributing to the Increase in the Number and Percent of Nonmarital Births

The combined factors of more unmarried women of childbearing age in the population and the increased birth rates of unmarried women resulted in dramatic increases in the *number* of nonmarital births over the last several decades. The text box shows that the percentage of women of childbearing age increased about 16% during the period from 1960 to 1990, from 39.7% to 46.0%. **Table 3** shows that the percent of women who never married increased from 11.9% in 1960 to 22.0% in 2006 (an 85% increase).

Table 2. Median Age at First Marriage, 1950-2006

Year	Men	Women
1950	22.8	20.3
1960	22.8	20.3
1970	23.2	20.8
1980	24.7	22.0
1990	26.1	23.9
1995	26.9	24.5
1996	27.1	24.8
1997	26.8	25.0
1998	26.7	25.0
1999	26.9	25.1
2000	26.8	25.1
2001	26.9	25.1
2002	26.9	25.3
2003	27.1	25.3
2004	27.4	25.3
2005	27.1	25.3
2006	27.5	25.5

Source: U.S. Census Bureau. Historical Time Series, Marital Status (MS-2), Family and Living Arrangements, 2008.

In addition, the *percent* of all births to unmarried women rose substantially over the last several decades as well. The reason for the increase was primarily due to three concurrent demographic factors. First, the number and proportion of unmarried women increased as more and more women from the baby boom generation postponed marriage.

PERCENT OF FEMALE POPULATION AGES 15-44
1960 39.7%
1970 40.7%
1980 45.4%
1990 46.0%
2000 42.9%
2006 41.0%

Postponement of Marriage

Since the 1960s, couples have postponed marriage. **Table 2** shows that in 1950 and 1960 the median age at first marriage was 22.8 years for men and 20.3 years for women. In 2006, for both men and women the median age at first marriage had increased by more than four years. An increasing share of men and women also have never been married. **Table 3** shows that in 1960, 11.9% of females age 15 and older (and 17.3% of males of the same age) had not yet married, compared to 22.0% of females (and 28.6% of males) in 2006.

The second demographic factor is that the birth rates for unmarried women of all ages continued to increase. Third, the birth rates for married women decreased. Thus, the percent of all births that were to unmarried women rose because births to unmarried women increased while births to married women decreased.[73]

Attitude Toward Marriage

During the last half-century, the median age at first marriage has increased for both men and women by more than four years. As seen in **Table 2**, in 2006, the median age at first marriage was 27.5 years for men and 25.5 years for women. Marriage postponement has increased the number of unmarried women in the population. In 2006, 22.0% of all females (ages 15 and older) had not yet married, the comparable figure in 1960 was 11.9% (see **Table 3**).[74]

Table 3. Percentage Distribution of Never Married Women, by Age, Selected Years 1960-2006

Age and Sex	1960	1970	1980	1990	1995	2000	2005	2006
Women (all)	11.9	13.7	17.1	18.9	19.4	21.1	21.6	22.0
15-19	NA	NA	NA	NA	NA	NA	NA	NA
20-24	28.4	35.8	50.2	62.8	66.8	72.8	74.6	75.3
25-29	10.5	10.5	20.9	31.1	35.3	38.9	41.3	43.1
30-34	6.9	6.2	9.5	16.4	19.0	21.9	23.6	24.0
35-39	6.1	5.4	6.2	10.4	12.6	14.3	15.6	16.7
40-44	6.1	4.9	4.8	8.0	8.7	11.8	12.1	13.1
45-54	7.0	4.9	4.7	5.0	6.1	8.6	9.7	10.3
55-64	8.0	6.8	4.5	3.9	4.3	4.9	6.1	6.5
65-74	8.5	7.8	5.6	4.6	4.0	3.7	4.1	3.9
75 and older	—	7.5	6.3	5.4	4.4	3.5	3.8	3.2

Source: U.S. Census Bureau, Statistical Abstract of the United States, 2007 and selected years.

Note: Although the (all) category represents the percentage of persons age 15 years and older who were never married, data for persons under age 20 are not available consistently for the selected years. Also, data for 1960 represent persons 65 years and older.

NA = Not available.

There is much agreement that the link between marriage and parenthood has weakened considerably. Many policymakers contend that the link must be firmly reestablished for the well-being of children and the good of the nation.[80]

Attitudes towards marriage are varied and complex. Fifty years ago, marriage was the central and defining feature of adult identity. It was intertwined with moral rightness. Although some viewed marriage as a form of social obligation and a restriction on personal freedom, it was considered the proper progression by most Americans.[75] Today, most Americans continue to view marriage as a natural stage in life. They also generally perceive marriage as a way toward personal growth and deeper intimacy. Some view it as a way to share one's life with someone in a committed loving relationship.[76] Others view it as a safe haven that imbues sexual faithfulness, emotional support, mutual trust, and lasting commitment.[77] Others are more cynical and view it as a relationship mainly designed for the sexual and emotional gratification of each adult.[78]

Although attitudes towards marriage have changed, most people eventually marry and the desire to marry is widespread. Generally, teens think that having a good marriage is important, and most say that it is likely they will get married. But they are less than certain that their future marriages will last a lifetime. In addition, marriage is facing stiff competition from cohabitation. Living together before getting married is considered acceptable by most young people.[79] Moreover, sex outside of marriage (especially for adults) is almost considered the norm and has virtually no stigma attached to it.

Lack of Marriageable Partners

The so-called shortage of "marriageable" men (both the number of unmarried men and the "quality" of unmarried men, as viewed in terms of their ability to support a family) has been cited as one explanation for declining marriage rates, and to a lesser extent for why nonmarital childbearing has increased.[81] In effect, although some women may have sexual relations with certain men, it does not mean that they consider those men to be viable marriage partners. A national survey of unmarried adults under age 35 found that more than two-thirds of the women surveyed and one-third of the men said that they would be "not at all willing to marry someone who was not likely to hold a steady job." This sentiment was shared across racial and ethnic groups.[82] Nonetheless, the "shortage of marriageable" men argument is primarily associated with black men and women. In *The Truly Disadvantaged,* William Julius Wilson argued that as rates of employment and rates of labor force participation dropped for young black men, the number of *desirable* marriage partners for black women also decreased.[83] In other words, many black women (and women generally) limit their marriage universe to men with steady jobs (and other desirable attributes).

Biological Clock Issues

Women may choose to have children outside of marriage because of concerns that they are older, unmarrried, and may no longer have the opportunity to have children. This is especially true among professional women who have pursued postsecondary education and have been entrenched in time-consuming careers. In addition, some women are not willing to sacrifice their independence or their desire to have children, simply for sake of marriage.[84] Since the 1990s, some women have used new technology such as in-vitro fertilization and sperm donation procedures to have a child without a spouse.

Cohabiting Relationships

In contrast to years past, today many children born outside of marriage are born to cohabiting parents rather than to biological parents who live in separate households. Nonetheless, it is generally agreed that cohabiting relationships are less stable than marriage. In 1977, there were 1.1 million family households (with children under age 18) that consisted of cohabiting couples. In 2007, 6.4 million family households (with children under age 18) consisted of cohabiting couples. Thus in that 30-year period, cohabiting couples as a share of all family households increased from 2% to 8.2%. According to one report: "Just as it has become more common for couples to have intercourse and to live together without marrying, it has become more likely that couples who conceive outside marriage will remain unmarried."[85]

Growing up with two continuously cohabiting biological parents is rare. The Fragile Families Study indicates that about one-fourth of cohabiting biological parents are no longer living together one year after the child's birth.[86] Another study of first births found that 31% of cohabiting couples had broken up after five years, as compared to 16% of married couples. A study using the 1999 National Survey of American Families found that only 1.5% of all children lived with two cohabiting parents at the time of the survey. Similarly, an analysis of the 1995 Adolescent Health Study revealed that less than one-half of 1% of adolescents ages 16 to 18 had spent their entire childhoods living with two continuously cohabiting biological parents.[87]

Divorce

If a woman is divorced and engages in sexual relations she may become pregnant and thereby may have a child outside of marriage. A recent study using cohort analysis found that 14.4% of nonmarital births were to women who had divorced but not yet remarried.[88] The discussion below briefly highlights trends in divorce, median duration of divorce, and proportions of women who remarry.

In 1950, the marriage rate was more than four times the divorce rate (11.1 per 1,000 population versus 2.6 per 1,000 population); by 2006, it was only twice the divorce rate (7.3 per 1,000 population versus 3.6 per 1,000 population). Although marriage and divorce data are usually displayed as rates, researchers generally agree that a comparison of marriage and divorce rates is misleading because the persons who are divorcing in any given year are typically not the same as those who are marrying.

In 2004, 23% of U.S. women who were once married had been divorced. The median duration of marriages before divorce was about 8 years. The median time between divorce and a second marriage was about three and a half years. In 2004, 12% of men and 13% of women had married twice, and 3% of both men and women had married three or more times. Among adults 25 and older who had ever divorced, 52% of men and 44% of women were currently married.[89]

Sexual Activity Outside of Marriage

Sexual activity outside of marriage is associated with nonmarital births. A study that was based on data from several panels of the National Survey of Family Growth found that, by age 44, 95% of those surveyed had engaged in sexual activity (intercourse) before marriage.[90] According to the survey, 69% of women ages 15 through 44 who had never been married and who were not cohabiting had engaged in sexual intercourse.[91] If in fact such a large percentage of unmarried men and women are engaging in sex they are at risk of becoming parents (unless their choice of contraception is effective).[92]

Risk factors and behaviors may contribute to the increase in sex outside of marriage among teenagers. A report on research findings on programs that attempt to reduce teen pregnancy and STDs contends that hundreds of factors affect teen sexual behavior. Among them are (1) community disorganization (violence and substance abuse are prevalent); (2) family disruption, including substance abuse by family members and physical abuse and general maltreatment; (3) the mother had a child at a young age; (4) an older sibling engaged in sex; (5) close friends are older; (6) friends drink alcohol and use drugs; (7) friends have permissive views regarding sex; (8) friends are sexually active; (9) the youth is romantically involved with someone older; (10) the youth has problems with understanding and completing schoolwork; (11) the youth uses alcohol and other drugs; (12) the youth is part of a gang; (13) the youth is frequently involved in fighting and has carried a weapon;

(14) the youth works more than 20 hours per week; (15) the youth has permissive attitudes toward premarital sex; (16) the youth dates frequently or is going steady; and (17) the girl has several boyfriends.[93] The author maintains that many of the risk factors and behaviors can be changed with effective youth development programs.[94]

Declining Abortion Rates

The decrease in the rate of abortions may contribute to the increasing share of unmarried women who have children. According to the Guttmacher Institute, nearly half of all pregnancies to American women are unintended. Moreover, about 20% of all pregnancies end with an abortion. The annual number of legal abortions in the United States increased through the 1970s, leveled off in the 1980s, dropped in the 1990s, and has continued to drop from 2000 through 2005. The number of abortions was 1.554 million in 1980, 1.609 million in 1990 (a record high), 1.313 million in 2000, 1.287 million in 2003, and 1.206 million in 2005.[95]

Women who have abortions tend to be unmarried and white, and a disproportionate share are in their twenties. In 2003 (latest available comprehensive data), about eight of ten females who had abortions were unmarried. White females (who represented about 80% of the U.S. female population in 2003) constituted 56% of the females who had abortions in 2003, followed by black and other women who had 44% of the abortions in 2003. Also in 2003, of those females who had abortions, the largest percentage was among women ages 20 through 24 (33%). The remaining shares were 1% for girls under age 15; 17% for women ages 15 through 19; 23% for women ages 25 through 29; 15% for women ages 30 through 34; 8% for women ages 35 through 39; and 3% for women age 40 or over. For nearly half (46%) of the women who had an abortion in 2003 it was not their first abortion.[96]

IMPACT OF NONMARITAL BIRTHS ON FAMILIES

Although 38.5% of all U.S. births in 2006 were to women who were not married, 23.3% of the 73.7 million U.S. children under age 18 lived in mother-only families in 2006.[97] The difference occurs because the proportion of births to unmarried women has increased over the past several decades and because some of these women married and some were in cohabiting relationships.[98]

A wide body of research indicates that children who grow up with only one biological parent in the home are more likely to be financially worse off and have worse socioeconomic outcomes (even after income differences are taken into account) compared to children who grow up with both biological parents in the home.[99] Specifically, children living in a single-parent home are more likely to do poorly in school, have emotional and behavioral problems, become teenage parents, and have poverty-level incomes (as children and adults) than children living with married biological parents.[100] Further, children in single-parent families are six times more likely to be poor than children in two-parent families. It has been reported that 22% of children in one-parent families will experience poverty during childhood for seven years or more, as compared to only 2% of children in two-parent families.[101] In 2007, 7.5% of children under age 18 living in married-couple families were living below the poverty level compared to 38.3% of children living with mother-only families.[102]

> One analyst makes the following assertion regarding two-parent families:
> Social science research is almost never conclusive. There are always methodological difficulties and stones left unturned. Yet in three decades of work as a social scientist, I know of few other bodies of data in which the weight of evidence is so decisively on one side of the issue: on the whole, for children, two-parent families are preferable to single-parent and stepfamilies.[103]

Others assert that although marriage of biological parents is associated with greater child well-being, little is known about why or how much of the relationship is caused by marriage and how much by other factors. In other words, it could be that the effect of marriage on child well-being is derived not from marriage itself, but rather from the distinctive characteristics of the individuals who marry and stay married (sometimes referred to as the "selection effect").[104] It is sometimes argued that some of the problems associated with non-intact families may be the effect of poverty rather than the father's absence. Further, most children who grow up in mother-only families or step-parent families become well-adjusted, productive adults. For some children, the absence of the father may result in freedom from an abusive or otherwise difficult situation and may result in a more supportive loving mother-child relationship.

IMPACT OF NONMARITAL BIRTHS ON THE NATION

This section reviews assertions that it is not just the family that is negatively affected by nonmarital childbearing, but the taxpayer as well. It discusses some of the impacts of financial and demographic factors associated with nonmarital births on the population as a whole.

Potential Financial Costs

Although the three reports mentioned below do not categorically say that nonmarital births cost the federal government a specific dollar amount, they do provide a context in which to consider the financial costs associated with nonmarital childbearing. The first report examines nonmarital childbearing and divorce together to measure taxpayer costs of what the author calls family fragmentation, but it does not separately attribute costs to nonmarital childbearing. The second study examines how poverty in the U.S. would be affected if more children were living in two-parent families. The third report attributes a specific dollar amount to the consequences of teens having children.

A 2008 report[105] examines the economic costs associated with the decline in marriage (which the authors contend increases the number of children and adults eligible for and in need of government services). The authors of the report maintain that the decline in marriage is a product of both divorce and unmarried childbearing. The report estimates that *combined*, the high rates of divorce and nonmarital childbearing costs U.S. taxpayers at least $112 billion per year in federal, state, and local costs — $70.1 billion of which is federal costs.[106] The report states that "These costs arise from increased taxpayer expenditures for antipoverty, criminal justice, and education programs, and through lower levels of taxes paid by individuals who, as adults, earn less because of reduced opportunities as a result of having been more likely to grow up in poverty."[107]

Another study examined the impact of nonmarital childbearing on poverty by using a regression approach that was based on hypothetically matching single women and men in the population on the basis of factors such as age, education, and race. It found that if the share of children living with two parents in 2000 was increased to what it had been in 1970, the child poverty rate in 2000 would have declined by about 29% compared to the actual decline of 4.5%.[108] If that analysis is applied to 2007 data, 3.7 million fewer children would be in poverty.[109]

In addition, a 2006 report quantified the costs of adolescent childbearing.[110] As noted earlier, births to teens represented 10% of all births and 23% of nonmarital births (2005 data). The report estimated that, in 2004, adolescent childbearing cost U.S. taxpayers about $9 billion per year.[111] Specific estimates cited were $2.3 billion in child welfare benefits; $1.9 billion in health care expenses; $2.1 billion in spending on incarceration (for the sons of women who had children as adolescents); and $6.3 billion in lost tax revenue because of lower earnings of the mothers, fathers, and children (when they were adults). Added to these cost figures are $3.6 billion in savings that result from the declines in births to teens.[112] Research indicates that teens who give birth are less likely to complete high school and go on to college, thereby reducing their potential for economic self-sufficiency. The research also indicates that the children of teens are more likely than children of older parents to experience problems in school and drop out of high school and, as adults, are more likely to repeat the cycle of teenage pregnancy and poverty. The 2006 report contends that if the teen birth rate had not declined between 1991 and 2004, the annual costs associated with teen childbearing would have been almost $16 billion (instead of $9 billion).[113] Although these data are interesting, it is important to remember that although 83% of births to teens are nonmarital births, adolescent childbearing is only a subset of nonmarital childbearing.

Demographic Impacts

Having the birth rate reach the replacement rate is generally considered desirable by demographers and sociologists because it means a country is producing enough young people to replace and support aging workers without population growth being so high that it taxes national resources.[114]

An examination of nonmarital births from a demographic perspective is perhaps the only analysis that does not view nonmarital births as a negative phenomenon. The nation's total fertility rate — the number of children the average woman would be expected to bear in her lifetime — has been below the replacement level since 1972.[115] The replacement rate is the rate at which a given generation can exactly replace itself. The fertility level required for natural replacement of the U.S. population is about 2.1 births per woman (i.e., 2,100 births per 1,000 women). The replacement rate was reached in 2006 for the first time in many years.[116]

Given that the marital birth rate has been decreasing over time, if the birth rate of unmarried women had begun to reverse itself, the U.S. population would cease growing (if the immigration factor is excluded).[117] From a geopolitical perspective, this means that those who support policies to lower nonmarital fertility do so at the risk of lowering overall U.S. fertility that has been hovering near replacement levels.[118] In the United States, non-Hispanic white women and Asian women 40 to 44 years old had fertility levels below the replacement level (1.8 and 1.7 births per woman, respectively). The fertility level of black women ages 40 to 44 (2.0 births per woman) did not differ statistically from the natural replacement level.[119] Hispanic women ages 40 to 44 had an average of 2.3 births and were the only group that exceeded the fertility level required for natural replacement of the U.S. population.[120]

Nonmarital births are also influencing other demographic shifts. On the basis of the fertility rate of women by racial and ethnic groups, by 2050, 54% of the U.S. population will consist of minority groups (i.e., Hispanics, blacks, American Indians, and Asians). Minorities, now roughly one-third of the U.S. population, are expected to become the majority in 2042, with the nation projected to be 54% minority in 2050. By 2023, minorities will represent more than half of all children.[121] By 2050, the Hispanic population is projected to nearly triple, and its share of the nation's total population is projected to double, from 15% to 30%. Thus, nearly one in three U.S. residents will be Hispanic.[122] (As mentioned earlier, in 2005, 48% of Hispanic births were nonmarital births.) The black population is projected to increase from 14% of the population in 2008 to 15% in 2050. The Asian population's share of the nation's population is expected to rise from 5.1% to 9.2%. Among the remaining race groups, American Indians and Alaska Natives are projected to rise from 1.6% to 2% of the total population. The Native Hawaiian and Other Pacific Islander population is expected to more than double, from 1.1 million to 2.6 million, representing about 0.6% in 2050. The number of people who identify themselves as being of two or more races is projected to more than triple, from 5.2 million to 16.2 million, representing almost 4% of the population in 2050. Non-Hispanic whites are projected to represent 46% of the total population, down from 66% in 2008.[123]

PUBLIC POLICY INTERVENTIONS

In recognition of the potential long-term consequences of nonmarital births, the federal government's strategy to nonmarital childbearing has been varied. The federal government acknowledges that an effective approach for teenagers may be inappropriate for older women. Some observers criticize women much farther along the age spectrum who have nonmarital births as being selfish and not looking long-range to what would be in the best interest of their offspring. Other observers counter, pointing out that it is not the unmarried, college-educated, thirty-somethingyear-olds with well-paying jobs who are worried that their time for having a child is running out that should be a concern. Rather it is the millions of women for whom single motherhood is the norm, who entrench themselves and their children in a less favorable economic lifestyle by having a child outside of a healthy marriage. Many of these women become mothers in their teenage years.

In order to address these two distinct groups of females, federal policy toward teens has primarily focused on pregnancy prevention programs, whereas federal policy toward older women has focused on healthy marriage programs. Income support programs, such as the Child Support Enforcement program and the Temporary Assistance for Needy Families (TANF) block grant program, that attempt to reduce or ameliorate negative financial consequences that are sometimes associated with nonmarital childbearing are available to mothers of all age groups.

This section discusses the public policy interventions (1) directed at teens, such as abstinence education programs, comprehensive sex education programs, and youth programs; (2) focused on adults, namely the healthy marriage programs and the responsible fatherhood programs (that usually include several components dealing with improving communication skills with respect to the other parent); and (3) provided to all persons regardless of age such as family planning programs, adoption services, and federal income support programs — the Child Support Enforcement and Temporary Assistance for Needy Families (TANF) programs.

Abstinence Promotion

Many argue that sexual activity in and of itself is wrong if the individuals are not married. Advocates of the abstinence education approach argue that teenagers need to hear a single, unambiguous message that sex outside of marriage is wrong and harmful to their physical and emotional health. These advocates contend that youth can and should be empowered to say no to sex. They argue that supporting both abstinence and birth control is hypocritical and undermines the strength of an abstinence-only message. They also cite research that indicates that teens who take virginity pledges to refrain from sex until marriage appear to delay having sex longer than those teens who do not make such a commitment. (One study found that teens who publicly promise to postpone sex until marriage refrain from intercourse for about a year and a half longer than teens who did not make such a pledge.)[124] They further argue that abstinence is the most effective (100%) means of preventing unwanted pregnancy and sexually transmitted diseases (including HIV/AIDS).[125]

Three federal programs include funding that is exclusively for abstinence education: Adolescent Family Life (AFL) program, the Title V Abstinence Education Block Grant to States, and the Community-Based Abstinence Education (CBAE) program.[126] All of these programs are carried out by the Department of Health and Human Services (HHS). For FY2008, federal abstinence education funding totaled $177 million: $13 million for AFL abstinence education projects; $50 million for the Title V Abstinence Education Block Grant to states; and $109 million for the CBAE program (up to $10 million of which may be used for a national abstinence education campaign); and $4.5 million for an evaluation of the CBAE program.[127]

The AFL demonstration program was enacted in 1981 as Title XX of the Public Health Service Act (P.L. 97-35). It is administered by the Office of Adolescent Pregnancy Programs at HHS. From 1981 until 1996, the AFL program was the only federal program that focused directly on the issues of adolescent sexuality, pregnancy, and parenting.[128] The AFL program was designed to promote family involvement in the delivery of services, adolescent premarital sexual abstinence, adoption as an alternative to early parenting, parenting and child development education, and comprehensive health, education, and social services geared to help the mother have a healthy baby and improve subsequent life prospects for both mother and child. The AFL program authorizes grants for three types of demonstrations: (1) projects that provide "care" services only (i.e., health, education, and social services to pregnant adolescents, adolescent parents, their infant, families, and male partners); (2) projects that provide "prevention" services only (i.e., services to promote abstinence from premarital sexual relations for pre-teens, teens, and their families); and (3) projects that provide a combination of care and prevention services. Any public or private nonprofit organization or agency is eligible to apply for a demonstration grant. AFL projects can be funded for up to five years.

The Title V Abstinence Education Block Grant to States was authorized under P.L. 104-193 (the 1996 welfare reform law). The law provided $50 million per year for five years (FY1998-FY2002) in federal funds specifically for the abstinence education program. Although the program has not yet been reauthorized, the latest extension, contained in P.L. 110-275, continues funding for the abstinence-only block grant through June 30, 2009. Funds must be requested by states when they solicit Title V Maternal and Child Health (MCH) block grant funds and must be used exclusively for teaching abstinence. To receive federal funds, a state must match every $4 in federal funds with $3 in state funds.[129] This means that full funding (from states and the federal government) for abstinence education must total at least $87.5 million annually.

Additional abstinence-only education funding, for the CBAE program,[130] has been included in appropriations measures. The program provides abstinence-only education for adolescents aged 12 through 18. Funding for the program increased incrementally, from $30 million in FY2002 to $109 million in FY2008.

Evaluation of Abstinence Education Programs

Mathematica's April 2007 report presents the final results from a multi-year, experimentally based impact study on several abstinence-only block grant programs. The report focuses on four selected Title V abstinence education programs for elementary and middle school students. On the basis of follow-up data collected from youth (aged 10 to 14) four to six years after study enrollment, the report, among other things, presents the estimated program impacts on sexual abstinence and risks of pregnancy and STDs. According to the report,

> Findings indicate that youth in the program group were no more likely than control group youth to have abstained from sex and, among those who reported having had sex, they had similar numbers of sexual partners and had initiated sex at the same mean age.... Program and control group youth did not differ in their rates of unprotected sex, either at first intercourse or over the last 12 months.... Overall, the programs improved identification of STDs but had no overall impact on knowledge of unprotected sex risks and the consequences of STDs. Both program and control group youth had a good understanding of the risks of pregnancy but a less clear understanding of STDs and their health consequences.[131]

In response to the report, HHS has stated that the Mathematica study showcased programs that were among the first funded by the 1996 welfare reform law. It stated that its recent directives to states have encouraged states to focus abstinence-only education programs on youth most likely to bear children outside of marriage, that is, high school students, rather than elementary or middle-school students. It also mentioned that programs need to extend the peer support for abstinence from the preteen years through the high school years.[132]

Comprehensive Sex Education

Advocates of a comprehensive approach to sex education argue that today's youth need information and decision-making skills to make realistic, practical decisions about whether to engage in sexual activities. They contend that such an approach allows young people to make informed decisions regarding abstinence, gives them the information they need to set relationship limits and to resist peer pressure, and also provides them with information on the use of contraceptives and the prevention of sexually transmitted diseases.[133] They argue that about 50% of high school students have experienced sexual intercourse.[134] They maintain that abstinence-only messages provide no protection against the risks of pregnancy and disease for those who are sexually active. They point out that, according to one study, teens who break their virginity pledges were less likely to use contraception the first time than teens who had never made such a promise.[135]

In addition, the alarming number of females under age 25 with sexually transmitted diseases (STDs)[136] has re-energized efforts to persuade girls and young women to abstain from sexual activity or to use condoms (along with other forms of contraceptives) to prevent or reduce pregnancy as well as reduce their risk of getting STDs.[137]

No earmarked federal funding currentlyexists for comprehensive sex education in schools. In other words, there is no federal appropriation specifically for comprehensive sex education. Although there is not a federal comprehensive sex education program per se, many federal programs provide information about contraceptives, provide contraceptive services to teens, and provide referral and counseling services related to reproductive health. These programs include Medicaid Family Planning, Title X FamilyPlanning, and Adolescent Family Life care services. Also, funds from the Maternal and

Child Health block grant, the Title XX Social Services block grant, and the TANF block grant can be used to provide contraceptive services to teens.[138]

Evaluation of Comprehensive Sex Education Programs

There have been numerous evaluations of teen pregnancy prevention programs, but most of them did not use a scientific approach with experimental and control groups — an approach that most analysts agree provides more reliable, valid, and objective information than other types of evaluations. A recent report by the National Campaign to Prevent Teen Pregnancy,[139] however, highlighted five teen pregnancy prevention programs that were subjected to a random assignment, experimentally designed study.[140] These five comprehensive sex education programs were found to be effective in delaying sexual activity, improving contraceptive use among sexually active teenagers, or preventing teen pregnancy.

Many analysts and researchers agree that effective pregnancy prevention programs: (1) convince teens that not having sex or that using contraception consistently and carefully is the right thing to do; (2) last a sufficient length of time; (3) are operated by leaders who believe in their programs and who are adequately trained; (4) actively engage participants and personalize the program information; (5) address peer pressure; (6) teach communication skills; and (7) reflect the age, sexual experience, and culture of young persons in the programs.[141]

Youth Programs

Youth programs generally include one or more of the following components to address teen sexual activity: sex education, mentoring and counseling, health care, academic support, career counseling, crisis intervention, sports and arts activities, and community volunteer experiences. Youth programs receive funding from a wide array of sources, including the federal government, state and local governments, community organizations, private agencies, nonprofit organizations, and faith-based organizations.

The sex education component of many youth programs usually includes an abstinence message (which enables teens to avoid pregnancy) along with discussions about the correct and consistent use of contraception (which reduces the risk of pregnancy for sexually active teens). There is a significant difference between abstinence as a *message* and abstinence-only *interventions*. Although the Bush Administration continues to support an abstinence-only program intervention (with some modifications), others argue that an abstinence message integrated into a comprehensive sex education program that includes information on the use of contraceptives and that enhances decision-making skills is a more effective method to prevent teen pregnancy. A recent nationally representative survey found that 90% of adults and teens agree that young people should get a strong message that they should not have sex until they are at least out of high school and that a majority of adults (73%) and teens (56%) want teens to get more information about both abstinence and contraception.[142] The American public — both adults and teens — support encouraging teens to delay sexual activity *and* providing young people with information about contraception.[143]

A study that evaluated youth programs that sought to delay the first time teens have sex partly summarized the research by highlighting some characteristics or activities associated with teenagers who delayed sexual activity. The study reported that (1) teens who do well in school and attend religious services are more likely to delay sexual initiation; (2) girls who participate in sports also delay sex longer than those who do not; and (3) teens whose friends have high educational aspirations, who avoid such risky behavior as drinking or using drugs, and who perform well in school are less likely to have sex at an early age than teens whose friends do not.[144]

Some youth programs have an underlying goal of trying to decipher the root reasons behind teen pregnancy and childbearing. Is it loneliness or trying to find love or a sense of family? Is it carelessness — not bothering with birth control or using it improperly — or shame — not wanting to go to the doctor to ask about birth control or not wanting to be seen in a pharmacy purchasing birth control? Is it a need to meet the sexual expectations of a partner? Is it trying to find individual independence or is it defiance (a mentality of you can't boss me or control me, "I'm grown")? Is it trying to validate or provide purpose to one's life? Is it realistically facing the probability that the entry-level job she can get at the age of 18 is the same or similar to the one she will likely have when she is 30, thus why should she wait to have a child?

In addition, many youth programs also want to prevent second or additional births to teens, and they realize that a different approach may be needed to prevent secondary births as compared to first births. Research has indicated that youth programs that include mentoring components, enhanced case management, home visits by trained nurses or program personnel, and parenting classes have been effective in reducing subsequent childbearing by teens.[145]

Healthy Marriage Programs

Much of the increase in nonmarital childbearing results from changes in marital behavior rather than changes in fertility behavior. In other words, Americans are not having more babies, they are having fewer marriages.[146] The first finding of P.L. 104-193 (the 1996 welfare reform law) is that marriage is the foundation of a successful society. The second finding is that marriage is an essential institution of a successful society that promotes the interests of children. The law sought to promote marriage through the new TANF program. As authorized by P.L. 104-193, the TANF program established as statutory goals to promote the formation and maintenance of two-parent families and to reduce welfare dependence via job preparation, work, and marriage. Pursuant to the law, states may spend TANF funds on a wide range of activities (services) for cash welfare recipients and other families toward the achievement of these goals.

P.L. 109-171 (the Deficit Reduction Act of 2005) established new categorical grants within TANF for healthy marriage promotion and responsible fatherhood initiatives.[147] The healthy marriage promotion initiative is funded at approximately $100 million per year (FY2006-FY2010), to be spent through grants awarded by HHS to support research and demonstration projects by public or private entities; and technical assistance provided to states, Indian tribes and tribal organizations, and other entities. The activities supported by the healthy marriage promotion initiatives are programs to promote marriage to the general population, such as public advertising campaigns on the value of marriage and education in high schools on the value of marriage; education on "social skills" (e.g., marriage education, marriage skills, conflict resolution, and relationship skills) for engaged couples, those interested in marriage, or married couples; and programs that reduce the financial disincentive to marry,[148] if combined with educational or other marriage promotion activities. Entities that apply for marriage promotion grants must ensure that participation in such activities is voluntary and that domestic violence concerns are addressed (e.g., through consultations with experts on domestic violence).[149]

Critics of healthy marriage programs caution that government must be careful about supporting programs that provide cash incentives to induce people to marry or that coerce or cajole individuals into marrying. They note the problems associated with child-bride marriages and the short-term and often unhappy nature of the so-called "shot-gun" marriage. Supporters of healthy marriage programs remark that many long-lasting marriages were based on financial alliances (e.g., to increase economic status, family wealth, status in the community, etc.). They assert that policies or programs designed to promote healthy marriages are not intended to force anyone into unwanted, unhealthy relationships, trap women in abusive relationships, or withdraw support from single mothers. Supporters maintain that a relationship is not healthy if it is not safe.

Nonetheless, many observers are concerned about the impact of healthy marriage promotion programs on survivors of domestic violence or those still in abusive relationships. They assert that all marriage promotion programs must identify and respond to domestic violence issues in a manner that is effective for the individual program in question.[150] Some observers contend that policymakers should focus healthy marriage programs on couples who want to get married, couples who are free from substance abuse problems and/or violent tendencies, and couples who do not have any children by other partners.[151]

Evaluation of Healthy Marriage Programs

HHS is sponsoring three multi-year impact evaluations of the Healthy Marriage program. Two of the three studies use a random assignment approach in which couples are assigned to either an experimental group (group that receives the program services) or a control group (group that does not receive program services). One study, called Building Strong Families, focuses on low-income unmarried parents. This study began in 2002 and is expected to continue through 2011; it is using an experimental design. A second study, called Supporting HealthyMarriages, focuses on low-income married parents, began in 2003 and is expected to continue through 2012; it is using an experimental design. A third study, called Community Healthy Marriage Initiative, focuses on families in three geographic communities (i.e., Milwaukee, Wisconsin; Dallas, Texas; and St. Louis, Missouri — with comparison communities (Cleveland, Ohio; Ft. Worth, Texas, and Kansas City, Missouri) where there are no federally funded healthy marriage programs. This third study began in 2003 and is expected to continue through 2011. A final report on the impact of each of the three programs is expected between 2011 and 2013.[152]

Responsible Fatherhood Programs

Connecting or reconnecting children to their noncustodial parents has become a goal of federal social policy. During the 106th Congress, then-Representative Nancy Johnson, chair of the Ways and Means Subcommittee on Human Resources, stated, "to take the next step in welfare reform we must find a way to help children by providing them with more than a working mother and sporadic child support." She noted that many low-income fathers have problems similar to those of mothers on welfare — namely, they are likely to have dropped out of high school, to have little work experience, and to have significant barriers that lessen their ability to find or keep a job. She also asserted that in many cases these men are "dead broke" rather than "dead beats" and that the federal government should help these noncustodial fathers meet both their financial and emotional obligations to their children.[153]

In hopes of improving the long-term outlook for children in single-parent families, federal, state, and local governments, along with public and private organizations, are supporting programs and activities that promote the financial and personal responsibility of noncustodial fathers to their children and increase the participation of fathers in the lives of their children. These programs have come to be known as "responsible fatherhood" programs. To help fathers and mothers meet their parental responsibilities, many policy analysts and observers support broad-based collaborative strategies that go beyond welfare and child support agencies and include schools, work programs, prison systems, churches, community organizations, and the health care system.

Most responsible fatherhood programs include media campaigns that emphasize the importance of emotional, physical, psychological, and financial connections of fathers to their children. Most fatherhood programs include parenting education; responsible decision-making; mediation services for both parents; providing an understanding of the CSE program; conflict resolution, coping with stress, and problem-solving skills; peer support; and job-training opportunities.

Although responsible fatherhood programs have been debated in Congress since the 106th Congress (1999) and supported from the start by the Bush Administration (2001), it was not until the Deficit Reduction Act of 2005 (P.L. 109-171, enacted February 8, 2006) was passed and enacted that specific funding was provided for responsible fatherhood programs.

P.L. 109-171 included a provision that provides up to $50 million per year (for each of the five fiscal years 2006-2010) in competitive grants through

TANF to states, territories, Indian tribes and tribal organizations, and public and nonprofit community organizations (including religious organizations) for responsible fatherhood initiatives. Under P.L. 109-171, responsible fatherhood funds can be spent on activities to promote responsible fatherhood through (1) marriage promotion (through counseling, mentoring, disseminating information about the advantages of marriage and two-parent involvement for children, etc.), (2) parenting activities (through counseling, mentoring, mediation, disseminating information about good parenting practices, etc.), (3) fostering economic stability of fathers (through work first services, job search, job training, subsidized employment, education, etc.), or (4) contracting with a nationally recognized nonprofit fatherhood promotion organization to develop, promote, or distribute a media campaign to encourage the appropriate involvement of parents in the lives of their children, particularly focusing on responsible fatherhood; and to develop a national clearinghouse to help states and communities in their efforts to promote and support marriage and responsible fatherhood.[154] According to data from the Administration for Children and Families (ACF) in the U.S. Department of Health and Human Services (HHS), 99 grantees were awarded five-year contracts to implement responsible fatherhood programs. The contracts (in aggregate) amounted to $41 million per year.[155]

Evaluation of Responsible Fatherhood Programs

Although Congress only recently authorized federal funding specifically earmarked for responsible fatherhood programs (via P.L. 109-171), many states and localities, private organizations, and nonprofit agencies have been operating responsible fatherhood programs for several years. Some researchers have noted that although there is a growing body of research on the impact of father absence in the lives of their children, there is not enough research on the benefits of father presence in the lives of their children. Several rather large demonstration projects have focused on noncustodial fathers, and this report highlights two of them.[156]

The Parents' Fair Share (PFS) Demonstration (designed and evaluated by MDRC) was a national demonstration project (that operated between 1994 and 1996) that combined job training and placement, peer support groups, and other services with the goal of increasing the earnings and child support payments of unemployed noncustodial parents (generally fathers) of children on welfare, improving their parenting and communication skills, and providing an opportunity for them to participate more fully and effectively in the lives of their children. The final report on the PFS demonstration concluded that the program did not significantly increase employment or earnings among the full sample of PFS participants during the two years after they entered the program. However, the program reportedly increased earnings among a subgroup of men who were characterized as "less employable" (i.e., those without a high school diploma and with little recent work experience).[157] Some analysts maintain that most of the fathers who participated in the PFS demonstration were estranged from their children when they entered the program and that some of them participated in lieu of serving time in jail. They assert that new unwed fathers are generally very attached to their children around the time of the child's birth and probably are more motivated than fathers of older children to take advantage of the opportunities or services offered by responsible fatherhood programs.[158]

The federal Office of Child Support Enforcement (OCSE) provided $2.0 million to fund Responsible Fatherhood demonstrations under Section 1115 of the Social Security Act. The programs operated in eight states between September 1997 and December 2002. The following eight states received Section 1115 grants or waivers from OCSE/Administration for Children and Families (ACF) to implement and test responsible fatherhood programs: California, Colorado, Maryland, Massachusetts, Missouri, New Hampshire, Washington, and Wisconsin. These projects attempted to improve the employment and earnings of under- and unemployed noncustodial parents, and to motivate them to become more financially and emotionally involved in the lives of their children. Although the projects shared common goals, they varied with respect to service components and service delivery. The outcome report found that employment rates and earnings increased significantly especially for noncustodial parents who were previously unemployed. In addition, child support compliance rates increased significantly especially for those who had not been paying previously. The report found that 27% of the fathers reported seeing their children more often after completion of the program.[159]

The outcome report on the OCSE Responsible Fatherhood programs also found that (1) low-income noncustodial fathers are a difficult population to recruit and serve; (2) many of the participants found jobs with the programs' help, but they were low-paying jobs, and relatively few of the participants were able to increase earnings enough to meet their financial needs and those of their children; (3) child access problems were hard to define and resolve, and mediation should be used more extensively; (4) child support guidelines result in orders for low-income noncustodial parents that are unrealistically high; (5) CSE agencies should collaborate with fatherhood programs and pursue routine enforcement activities, as well as adopt policies and incentives that are responsive to low-income fathers; and (6) criminal history was the norm rather than the exception among the program participants, many participants faced ongoing alcohol and substance abuse problems, many did not have reliable transportation, and many lacked a court-ordered visitation arrangement.[160]

Although several new evaluations are underway to scientifically determine whether responsible fatherhood programs work, they are many years from impact findings. Most are still at the initial stage of providing information on the implementation of the responsible fatherhood programs. An HHS-sponsored evaluation of responsible fatherhood programs, called the National Evaluation of the Responsible Fatherhood, Marriage and Family Strengthening Grants for Incarcerated and Re-entering Fathers and Their partners (MFS-IP), began in 2006 and is still enrollingparticipants. The evaluation is a multi-year (quasi-experimental) studythat is expected to run from 2006 through 2013. A final report on the impact of the program is expected between 2011 and 2013.[161]

Family Planning Services

One of the purposes of family planning services is to prevent unwanted pregnancies that may lead to nonmarital births. The National Family Planning Program, created in 1970 as Title X of the Public Health Service Act, is administered through the Office of Population Affairs/Office of Public Health and Science at HHS. It provides grants to public and private non-profit agencies to provide voluntary family planning services for individuals who are otherwise ineligible for medical services. Family planning programs provide basic reproductive health services: contraceptive services and supplies; infertility services; natural family planning methods education; special services to adolescents; adolescent abstinence counseling; gynecological care; screening for breast and cervical cancers; STD and HIV prevention education, counseling, and referrals; and reproductive health counseling, education, and referrals.

Priority for the provision of these services is to be given to lower-income families; grantees may use a sliding fee schedule for determining client contributions for care, but grantees may not charge low-income persons for care. The services must be provided "without coercion and with respect for the privacy, dignity, social, and religious beliefs of the individuals being served."[162]

Adoption

Some have said that adoption makes nonmarital childbearing "less visible" and perhaps to some more acceptable.[163] Mothers who place their infant for adoption are more likely to finish school and less likely to live in poverty. Further, mothers who choose to give up their infants for adoption are more likely to marry than those who parent their baby.[164]

Although adoption is not an intervention to negate nonmarital childbearing, it does present an alternative living arrangement for children born to unmarried parents. Adoption is the legal process of adding a person to an existing family. Adoption, unlike foster care, is meant to be permanent. The goal of adoption is to provide lifelong security to the child. According to some studies, children placed in adoptive homes have better scores in school and engage in less delinquent behavior than children raised by a single parent.[165]

"Shotgun" marriages and adoption were once viewed as the common remedies for a nonmarital birth. Even so, historically, adoption has played a very limited role as an alternative to mother-only families. Adoption has been and remains rare. There were approximately 130,000 adoptions in the U.S. in 2002.[166] Of these 130,000, the number that are children born to unmarried women is not known.[167]

Some observers contend that adoption might be viewed as a more viable option for an unwanted pregnancy if school systems included a meaningful discussion of adoption in their sex education classes.[168]

Child Support Obligation as a Deterrent

The Child Support Enforcement (CSE) program was enacted in 1975 as a federal-state program (Title IV-D of the Social Security Act) to help strengthen families by securing financial support for children from their noncustodial parent on a consistent and continuing basis and by helping some families to remain self-sufficient and off public assistance by providing the requisite CSE services. Over the years, CSE has evolved into a multifaceted program. Although cost-recovery still remains an important function of the program, its other aspects include service delivery and promotion of self-sufficiency and parental responsibility.

The CSE program contains numerous measures to establish and enforce child support obligations.[169] Because strict child support enforcement is thought to deter nonmarital childbearing, the child support provisions are seen by some in Congress as another method of attempting to reduce nonmarital pregnancies. Child support enforcement measures include streamlined efforts to name the father in every case, employer reporting of new hires (to locate noncustodial parents quicker), uniform interstate child support laws, computerized statewide collections to expedite payment, and stringent penalties, such as the revocation of a drivers' license and the seizure of bank accounts, in cases in which noncustodial parents owe past-due child support.

According to social science research, stronger child support enforcement may increase the cost of children for men and should make men more reluctant to have children outside of marriage. In other words, by raising the cost of fatherhood to unmarried men, effective paternity establishment and child support enforcement deter nonmarital births.[170] In contrast, stronger child support enforcement may reduce the cost of children for women (making them more willing to have children outside of marriage).[171] However, according to recent evidence, once a single woman becomes a mother, her chances of marrying anyone other than the father of her child are greatly reduced.[172]

Temporary Assistance for Needy Families (TANF): Title IV-A of the Social Security Act

The TANF block grant (Title IV-A of the Social Security Act) funds a wide range of benefits and services for low-income families with children. TANF was created by P.L. 104-193 (the 1996 welfare reform law). Its funding was extended through FY2010 by P.L. 109-171 (the Deficit Reduction Act of 2005, enacted February 8, 2006). One of the four goals of the 1996 welfare reform law (P.L. 104193) is to prevent and reduce out-of-wedlock pregnancies.[173] To this end, unmarried minor parents may only receive TANF assistance if they live at home or in an adult-supervised setting and attend school if they lack a high school diploma.

States are using TANF funds to support activities that may prevent nonmarital pregnancies. Generally these activities focus on preventing teen pregnancy. These activities are often classified as "youth services" (includes after-school programs for teens and sub-grants to community organizations such as Boys and Girls Clubs). Several states have reported that they conduct home visits to new parents, in an effort to reduce subsequent pregnancies. Many states reported operating abstinence education programs (which maybe funded in whole or in part through TANF or other federal abstinence education programs). In addition, family planning services can be funded in part from TANF or other federal grant programs.[174]

Another one of the four TANF goals is to promote the formation and maintenance of two-parent families. States have separate funding via their TANF programs to operate responsible fatherhood programs and marriage promotion initiatives (discussed below).

FUTURE PROSPECTS

The language regarding births to unmarried women has changed in significant ways. What once were referred to as "bastard" or "illegitimate" children are now termed "out-of-wedlock," "outside of marriage," or "nonmarital" births. The stigma and shame that had once been attached to these children is no longer recognized by the public.[175] Further, some commentators argue that the facts have been twisted in such a way that mothers are justified in having a nonmarital birth and that having a baby without a husband represents a higher level of maternal devotion and sacrifice than having a baby with a husband.[176] They assert that it is often the case that adults pursue individual happiness in their private relationships, which is in direct conflict with the needs of children for stability, security, and permanence in their family lives.[177]

Some observers contend that the problem is not the weakening of marriage (about 75% of all women ages 15 and older eventually marry), but rather the de-linking of marriage and having children and the abdication of the traditional view of marriage as a life-long commitment.[178] Some researchers and policymakers argue that although couple relationships are a private matter, an overwhelming body of evidence suggests that not all family structures produce equal outcomes for children. They maintain that there is widespread agreement that a healthy, stable (i.e., low-conflict) family with two biological parents is the best environment for children.[179] Finally, some observers assert that we as a society have not strayed too far, and that it is not too late to return to the somewhat old-fashioned, but not simplistic, precept of falling in love, getting married, and having a baby, in that order.[180]

Although marriage and family life are generally considered private issues, they have become part of the public arena primarily because of public policies that help families affected by negative outcomes associated with nonmarital births to maintain a minimum level of economic sufficiency.[181] The abundance of research on the subject of the impact on children of various living environments also raises the stakes — in that it is now almost unanimously agreed that children living with both biological parents fare better on a host of measures — economic, social, psychological, and emotional — than children living with a single parent or in a stepparent or cohabiting situation.[182]

One of the things that this report highlights is that although there has been a rise in nonmarital births, it does not mean that there has been a subsequent rise in mother-only families. Instead, it reflects the rise in the number of couples who are in cohabiting relationships. Because the number of women living in a cohabiting situation has increased substantially over the last several decades, many children start off in households in which both of their biological parents reside. Nonetheless, cohabiting family situations are disrupted or dissolved much more frequently than married-couple families.

As discussed in an earlier section, the federal government funds a number of programs that seek to (1) reduce or eliminate nonmarital childbearing or (2) ameliorate some of the negative outcomes often associated with children of unmarried parents. The rest of this section highlights several interventions that may receive further attention and more debate in Congress. Although this report does not base the analysis of increased nonmarital childbearing by segmenting teen births from other births, it is important to note that more than half of *first* nonmarital births are to teens. This means that policies that are successful in reducing births to teenagers would significantly lessen the problem of nonmarital childbearing.

The difference between the average age of first intercourse (seventeen) and the age at first marriage (twenty-five) for women is eight years. For the majority of adult women, living without a married spouse does not mean living without sex,[183] nor in many cases does it mean living without having children. In 2005, almost 20% of the women ages 40 and older who gave birth had a child born outside of marriage. For women ages 20 through 24, the percentage was almost 60%. These figures reflect the new paradigm of women in all age groups, not just teenagers, having children outside of marriage. Some observers and analysts assert that new strategies that account for this new paradigm must be developed to significantly reduce nonmarital births. Others argue that the nation must decide whether to try to change the fertility behavior of women in their thirties and forties. They contend that given the new economic framework and the scarcity of resources in most areas of public finance, it may be wiser to pursue a strategy that focuses primarily on adolescents and women in their early twenties.

Given the patterns of swift transitions into and out of marriage and the high rate of single parenthood, a family policy that relies too heavily on marriage will not help the many children who will live in single-parent and cohabiting families — many of them poor — during most of their formative years.[184] Moreover, national data from the 2002 panel of the National Survey of Family Growth indicate that 14% of white men, 32% of black men, and 15% of Hispanic men had children with more than one woman.[185] Thus, children in the same family may potentially face different outcomes. For example, children with the same mother and different fathers may potentially face less desirable outcomes if their mother marries the biological father of their half-brothers or half-sisters.[186]

The advantages married couples and their children have over those in other living arrangements led the Bush Administration and Congress to propose marriage promotion initiatives. The knowledge that American society has changed in ways that will no longer permit all children to live with their biological parents led the Bush Administration and Congress to support responsible fatherhood programs. Both the healthy marriage programs and the responsible fatherhood programs were funded by the same legislation (i.e., P.L. 109-171 under the auspices of the TANF block grant program).[187] The rationale for implementing these two approaches in a complementary manner was to promote the best interest of children.[188]

Although there was some animosity between proponents of healthy marriage programs and proponents of responsible fatherhood programs[189] when they were debated during the period from 2001 through 2005, there is a growing consensus that the two programs can be implemented in a complementary manner to promote the best interest of children.[190] Some of the impact analysis on the two programs, based on scientifically designed evaluations with experimental and control groups, is to be completed during the next Congress. This may help the 111th Congress and the new Administration to determine whether or not they need to shift priorities between the programs, redistribute funding, or make other changes that will improve the effectiveness of both programs.

Similarly, there is now some discussion about a middle ground between abstinence education and comprehensive sex education.[191] Some call this approach abstinence-plus. Under the abstinence-plus education approach, participants are given a hierarchy of safe-sex strategies. At the top of the hierarchy is the promotion of sexual abstinence as the safest route to pregnancy prevention and HIV and STD prevention. Recognizing that some participants will not be abstinent, the abstinence-plus approach encourages individuals to use condoms and to adopt other safer-sex strategies.[192] Proponents of the abstinence-plus approach contend that it does not encourage teens or young adults to have more sex, it just encourages them to do so safely if they do have sex. Some policymakers maintain that this middle ground approach accepts the reality that sexual activity among older teens and young adults is an entrenched by-product of today's society. They argue that it is not bad policy but rather good planning to educate persons who thought they would remain abstinent until marriage, but do not, with the appropriate information regarding contraceptive methods. They contend that an abstinence-plus education approach is in the best interest of young people and in the best interest of the nation.

As mentioned earlier, no federal funding is specifically earmarked for comprehensive sex education. Some observers contend that the debate over abstinence-only education versus comprehensive sex education will likely continue for several more years. They surmise that the issue of which approach is more appropriate and more effective for adolescents and older teens may receive renewed attention by the 111th Congress and the new Administration. They also note that the abstinence-plus approach may be further scrutinized within the context of the debate on abstinence-only versus comprehensive sex education.

APPENDIX A. DATA TABLE

Table A-1. Number, Percent, and Rate of Births to Unmarried Women and Birth Rate for Married Women, 1940-2006

	Number of Births To Unmarried Women	Percent of Births To Unmarried Women	Birth Rate per 1,000 Unmarried Women Ages 15-44	Birth Rate per 1,000 Married Women Ages 15-44
1940	89,500	3.8	7.1	NA
1941	95,700	3.8	7.8	NA
1942	95,500	3.4	8.0	NA
1943	98,100	3.3	8.3	NA

Table A-1. (Continued)

	Number of Births To Unmarried Women	Percent of Births To Unmarried Women	Birth Rate per 1,000 Unmarried Women Ages 15-44	Birth Rate per 1,000 Married Women Ages 15-44
1944	105,200	3.8	9.0	NA
1945	117,400	4.3	10.1	NA
1946	125,200	3.8	10.9	NA
1947	131,900	3.6	12.1	NA
1948	129,700	3.7	12.5	NA
1949	133,200	3.7	13.3	NA
1950	141,600	4.0	14.1	141.0
1951	146,500	3.9	15.1	NA
1952	150,300	3.9	15.8	NA
1953	160,800	4.1	16.9	NA
1954	176,600	4.4	18.7	NA
1955	183,300	4.5	19.3	153.7
1956	193,500	4.7	20.4	NA
1957	201,700	4.7	21.0	NA
1958	208,700	5.0	21.2	NA
1959	220,600	5.2	21.9	NA
1960	224,300	5.3	21.6	156.6
1961	240,200	5.6	22.7	155.8
1962	245,100	5.9	21.9	150.8
1963	259,400	6.3	22.5	145.9
1964	275,700	6.9	23.0	141.8
1965	291,200	7.7	23.4	130.2
1966	302,400	8.4	23.3	123.6
1967	318,100	9.0	23.7	118.7
1968	339,200	9.7	24.3	116.6
1969	360,800	10.0	24.8	118.8
1970	398,700	10.7	26.4	121.1
1971	401,400	11.3	25.5	113.2
1972	403,200	12.4	24.8	100.8
1973	407,300	13.0	24.3	94.7

	Number of Births To Unmarried Women	Percent of Births To Unmarried Women	Birth Rate per 1,000 Unmarried Women Ages 15-44	Birth Rate per 1,000 Married Women Ages 15-44
1974	418,100	13.2	23.9	94.2
1975	447,900	14.3	24.5	92.1
1976	468,100	14.8	24.3	91.6
1977	515,700	15.5	25.6	94.9
1978	543,900	16.3	25.7	93.6
1979	597,800	17.1	27.2	96.4
1980	665,747	18.4	29.4	97.0
1981	686,605	18.9	29.5	96.0
1982	715,227	19.4	30.0	96.2
1983	737,893	20.3	30.3	93.6
1984	770,355	21.0	31.0	93.1
1985	828,174	22.0	32.8	93.3
1986	878,477	23.4	34.2	90.7
1987	933,013	24.5	36.0	90.0
1988	1,005,299	25.7	38.5	90.8
1989	1,094,169	27.1	41.6	91.9
1990	1,165,384	28.0	43.8	93.2
1991	1,213,769	29.5	45.0	89.6
1992	1,224,876	30.1	44.9	88.5
1993	1,240,172	31.0	44.8	86.1
1994	1,289,592	32.6	46.2	82.9
1995	1,253,976	32.2	44.3	82.6
1996	1,260,306	32.4	43.8	82.3
1997	1,257,444	32.4	42.9	82.7
1998	1,293,567	32.8	43.3	84.2
1999	1,308,560	33.0	43.3	84.8
2000	1,347,043	33.2	44.1	87.4
2001	1,349,249	33.5	43.8	86.7
2002	1,365,966	34.0	43.7	86.3
2003	1,415,995	34.6	44.9	88.1
2004	1,470,189	35.8	46.1	87.6
2005	1,527,034	36.9	47.5	87.3
2006	1,641,700	38.5	50.6	NA

Source: U.S. Department of Health and Human Services, National Center for Health Statistics, "Nonmarital Childbearing in the United States, 1940-99," *National Vital Statistics Reports*, vol. 48, no. 16 (October 18, 2000). See also *National Vital Statistics Reports*, vol. 56, no. 6 (December 5, 2007). Birth rates for married mothers data are from — National Center for Health Statistics, Vital Statistics of the United States, 1994, vol. I, Natality, Table 1-19.

NA = Not available.

End Notes

[1] Kristin A. Moore, "Nonmarital Childbearing in the United States," Child Trends, Inc. in U.S. Department of Health and Human Services, National Center for Health Statistics, "Report to Congress on Out-of-Wedlock Childbearing," Executive Summary, September 1995 [DHHS pub. no. (PHS) 95-1257-1], p. 6.

[2] The Census Bureau data do not indicate the number of newborns by the marital status of their parents, but data are available for children under age one by parents' marital status. In 2007, 59.4% of the 1.038 million children under age one were living with their biological mothers who had never married, 3.4% were living with their biological fathers who had never married, and 37.2% were living with both biological parents who were not married to each other. Source: U.S. Census Bureau, *America's Families and Living Arrangements: 2007*, Table C3.

[3] Sara McLanahan and Gary Sandefur, "Growing Up With a Single Parent: What Hurts, What Helps" (Cambridge, MA: Harvard University Press, 1994); see also L. Bumpass, "Children and Marital Disruption: A Replication and Update," *Demography*, vol. 21(1984), pp. 71-82.

[4] Marcia Carlson, Sara McLanahan, and Paula England, "Union Formation and Dissolution in Fragile Families," Fragile Families Research, Center for Research on Child Wellbeing, Princeton University, August 2002.

[5] Steven L. Nock, "Marriage as a Public Issue," *The Future of Children*, vol. 15, no. 2 (Fall 2005), p. 26.

[6] The sources of data for this report are varied. They primarily consist of (1) birth data from the National Center for Health Statistics at the Department of Health and Human Services (HHS), (2) income and poverty data from the Census Bureau, and (3) data on economic and demographic factors from the Fragile Families and Child Well-being Study and the 2002 panel of the National Survey of Family Growth.

[7] Kristin A. Moore, "Nonmarital Childbearing in the United States," Child Trends, Inc. in U.S. Department of Health and Human Services, National Center for Health Statistics, "Report to Congress on Out-of-Wedlock Childbearing," Executive Summary, September 1995 [DHHS pub. no. (PHS) 95-1257-1], p. 6.

[8] This report often uses the term women in describing data that include females who are under age 18.

[9] Elizabeth Terry-Humen, Jennifer Manlove, and Kristen A. Moore, "Births Outside of Marriage: Perception vs. Reality," Research Brief, *Child Trends*, April 2001.

[10] Sexual Behavior of Single Adult American Women, by Laura Duberstein Lindberg and Susheela Singh. *Perspectives on Sexual and Reproductive Health,* vol. 40., no. 1. March 2008.

[11] Sara McLanahan and Gary Sandefur, "Growing Up With a Single Parent: What Hurts, What Helps" (Cambridge, MA: Harvard University Press, 1994); see also L. Bumpass, "Children and Marital Disruption: A Replication and Update," *Demography*, vol. 21(1984), pp. 71-82;

see also Rebecca A. Maynard, ed., "Kids Having Kids: A Robin Hood Foundation Special Report on the Costs of Adolescent Childbearing" (New York, 1996); see also Mary Parke, "Are Married Parents Really Better for Children? What Research Says About the Effects of Family Structure on Child Well-Being," *Center for Law and Social Policy* (May 2003).

[12] Andrea Kane and Daniel T. Lichter, "Reducing Unwed Childbearing: The Missing Link in Efforts to Promote Marriage," *Center on Children and Families*, Brief no. 37 (April 2006).

[13] Daniel T. Lichter and Deborah Roempke Graefe, "Men and Marriage Promotion: Who Marries Unwed Mothers?," *Social Science Review* (September 2007).

[14] U.S. Census Bureau News. CB08-123. *An Older and More Diverse Nation by Midcentury.* August 14, 2008. Note: Non-Hispanic whites are projected to represent 46% of the total population in 2050, down from 66% in 2008. The black population is projected to increase from 14% of the population in 2008 to 15% in 2050. The Asian population is expected to rise from 5.1% to 9.2%. Among the remaining race groups, American Indians and Alaska Natives are projected to rise from 1.6% to 2% of the total population. The Native Hawaiian and Other Pacific Islander population is expected to more than double, from 1.1 million to 2.6 million, comprising about 0.6% in 2050. The number of people who identify themselves as being of two or more races is projected to more than triple, from 5.2 million to 16.2 million, representing almost 4% of the population in 2050.

[15] Even though one of the underlying purposes of this report is to discern why women get pregnant outside of marriage, this report solely uses birth data rather than pregnancy data. The reason for this is that birth data are more current and reliable than pregnancy data. Because of the difficulty in gathering the abortion and miscarriage data needed to calculate pregnancy data, pregnancy data lag about two to three years behind birth data reports.

[16] The proportion (i.e., percent) of births that occur to unmarried women is sometimes referred in the literature as the nonmarital birth ratio.

[17] The nonmarital birth rate during this period ranged from 42.9 to 44.3 births per 1,000 unmarried women ages 15-44.

[18] The nonmarital birth rate for all women in 2006 was 50.6 births per 1,000 unmarried women. The segmentation of the nonmarital birth rate by race and Hispanic origin for 2006 has not yet been published.

[19] The percentage of all U.S. births that were to unmarried women was 38.5% in 2006. The segmentation of the percentage of nonmarital births by race and Hispanic origin for 2006 is shown in **Table 1**.

[20] The text in this section discusses 2005 data because comparable 2006 nonmarital birth data on rates and numbers by race and ethnicity have not yet been published.

[21] Moynihan's 1965 report argued that black Americans were being held back economically and socially primarily because their family structure was deteriorating. The report was very controversial and sparked decades of debate. It was not until the 1990s that there was widespread agreement that Moynihan's prognostications were generally true.

[22] With respect to these statistics, "unmarried" is defined as being divorced, widowed, or never-married. The figures were calculated on the basis of data from the Census Bureau — America's Families and Living Arrangements: 2005 (males ages 15 and above and females ages 15 and above, by race and ethnicity), Table A1.

[23] Some commentators contend that in order for black women to find desirable marriage partners they may have to consider men of other races or cultures (e.g., African, Carribean).

[24] "Teenage Motherhood and Marriage," *Child Trends* and the *National Campaign to Prevent Teen Pregnancy.*

[25] Karen Benjamin Guzzo, "Multipartnered Fertility Among Young Women With a Nonmarital First Birth: Prevalence and Risk Factors," *Perspectives on Sexual and Reproductive Health,* March 2007.

[26] The Guttmacher Institute, "Teen Pregnancy: Trends and Lessons Learned," *The Guttmacher Report on Public Policy*, vol. 5, no. 1 (February 2002).

[27] In 2005, 23% of nonmarital white (non-Hispanic), black, and Hispanic births were to teenagers (under age 20); 25% of nonmarital American Indian/Alaskan Native and 16% of nonmarital Asian/Pacific Islander births were to teens (under age 20).

[28] U.S. Department of Health and Human Services, National Center for Health Statistics, "Births: Final Data for 2005," *National Vital Statistics Reports*, vol. 56, no. 6 (December 5, 2007).

[29] Elizabeth Terry-Humen, Jennifer Manlove, and Kristen A. Moore, "Births Outside of Marriage: Perception vs. Reality, Research Brief," *Child Trends*, April 2001.

[30] "Social Ecological Predictors of Repeat Adolescent Pregnancy,"*Perspectives on Sexual and Reproductive Health* (March 1, 2007).

[31] As mentioned earlier in the report, many women who have nonmarital births in their twenties first became mothers in their teen years. Thus, some observers contend that if teen pregnancy prevention programs were more effective, there would be fewer nonmarital births.

[32] Michael E. Foster and Saul D. Hoffman, "Nonmarital Childbearing in the 1980s: Assessing the Importance of Women 25 and Older," *Family Planning Perspectives*, (May/June 1996). See also Barbara Dafoe Whitehead, "Dan Quayle Was Right," *The Atlantic* (April 1993).

[33] Andrea Kane and Daniel T. Lichter, "Reducing Unwed Childbearing: The Missing Link in Efforts to Promote Marriage," *Center on Children and Families*, Brief no. 37 (April 2006). See also Paul R. Amato and Rebecca A. Maynard, "Decreasing Nonmarital Births and Strengthening Marriage to Reduce Poverty," *The Future of Children*, vol. 17, no. 2 (Fall 2007).

[34] Andrew J. Cherlin, "American Marriage in the Early Twenty-First Century," *The Future of Children*, vol. 15, no. 2 (Fall 2005), p. 38.

[35] Ibid., Table FG6.

[36] Lawrence L. Wu, Larry L. Bumpass, and Kelly Musick, "Historical and Life Course Trajectories of Nonmarital Childbearing," University of Wisconsin-Madison. *Center for Demography and Ecology*, Working Paper no. 99-23 (revised July 2000), p. 28.

[37] Elizabeth Terry-Humen, Jennifer Manlove, and Kristin A. Moore, "Births Outside of Marriage: Perceptions vs. Reality," Research Brief, *Child Trends*, April 2001.

[38] In 2007, 54% of mother-only families had one child, 31% had two children, 11% had three children, and 4% had four or more children. Source: U.S. Census Bureau, "America's Families and Living Arrangements: 2007," Table FG6.

[39] This means that the householder was living with someone of the opposite sex who was identified as his or her unmarried partner.

[40] This percentage is generally considered a low estimate because only householders and their partners (not all unmarried couples present in a household) are counted. In addition, some respondents may not want to admit that they are cohabiting and may instead described themselves as roommates, housemates, or friends.

[41] U.S. Census Bureau. Current Population Survey and Annual Social and Economic Supplements. July 2008.

[42] Larry Bumpass and Hsien-Hen Lu, "Trends in Cohabitation and Implications for Children's Family Contexts in the United States," *Population Studies*, vol. 54, no. 1 (March 2000), p. 29-41.

[43] Elizabeth Terry-Humen, Jennifer Manlove, and Kristin A. Moore, "Births Outside of Marriage: Perceptions vs. Reality," Research Brief, *Child Trends*, April 2001.

[44] Marcia Carlson, Sara McLanahan, and Paula England, "Union Formation in Fragile Families," *Demography* vol. 41 (2004), p. 237-61.

[45] Bumpass, Larry and Lu, Hsien-Hen(2000). "Trends in Cohabitation and Implications for Children's Family Contexts in the United States." *Population Studies*, 54: 29-41.

[46] U.S. Census Bureau, American Community Survey 2006, August 2008, Table 8.

[47] U.S. Census Bureau, America's Families and Living Arrangements: 2007, Tables F1 and UC3.

[48] U.S. Census Bureau, Current Population Survey and Annual Social and Economic Supplements, July 2008, Table F1.

[49] Elizabeth Terry-Humen, Jennifer Manlove, and Kristin A. Moore, "Births Outside of Marriage: Perceptions vs. Reality," Research Brief, *Child Trends*, April 2001. Also see U.S. Census Bureau, "America's Families and Living Arrangements 2000," P20-537 (June 2001), p. 13.

[50] U.S. Department of Health and Human Services. Centers for Disease Control and Prevention. National Survey of Family Growth. Fact Sheet. The percentages mentioned in the text are based on 2002 data and were limited to the first births of the mother. April 2008.

[51] Musick, Kelly, "Cohabitation, Nonmarital Childbearing, and the Marriage Process," *Demographic Research* [Germany], vol. 16, article 9 (April 20, 2007), p. 251.

[52] Jean Tansey Knab, "Cohabitation: Sharpening a Fuzzy Concept,"Center for Research on Child Wellbeing, Working Paper # 04-05-FF, May 2005, p. 2.

[53] Dore Hollander, "Nonmarital Childbearing in the United States: A Government Report," *Family Planning Perspectives*, vol. 28, no. 1 (January-February 1996), p. 32.

[54] Daniel T. Lichter and Deborah Roempke Graefe, "Finding a Mate? The Marital and Cohabitation Histories of Unwed Mothers," (November 1999), p. 9. Note: Some analysts contend that nonmarital fertility may be a behavioral manifestation of difficulties in finding a suitable marriage partner. The authors, based on their research, contend that nonmarital fertility has been a cause of the retreat from marriage. (Ibid, p. 4).

[55] Deborah Roempke Graefe and Daniel T. Lichter, "Marriage Among Unwed Mothers: Whites, Blacks and Hispanics Compared," *Perspectives on Sexual and Reproductive Health*, vol. 34, no. 6 (November/December 2002), p. 289.

[56] Andrea Kane and Daniel T. Lichter, "Reducing Unwed Childbearing: The Missing Link in Efforts to Promote Marriage," *Center on Children and Families*, Brief no. 37 (April 2006).

[57] George A. Akerlof, Janet L. Yellen and Michael L. Katz, "An Analysis of Out-of-Wedlock Childbearing in the United States," *The Quarterly Journal of Economics*, vol. 111, no. 2 (May 1996).

[58] Steven L. Nock and Christopher J. Einolf, "The One Hundred Billion Dollar Man: The Annual Public Costs of Father Absence," *The National Fatherhood Initiative* (June 2008) The federal programs include the Earned Income Tax Credit, TANF, CSE, Supplemental Security Income, Food Stamps, Special Program for Women, Infants, and Children (WIC), School Lunch, Medicaid, State Children's Health Insurance Program (SCHIP), Head Start, Child Care, Energy Assistance, Public Housing, and Section 8 Housing.

[59] Gladys M. Martinez, Anjani Chandra, Joyce C. Abma, Jo Jones, and William D. Mosher, "Fertility, Contraception, and Fatherhood: Data on Men and Women from Cycle 6 (2002) of the National Survey of Family Growth," Centers for Disease Control and Prevention, *National Center for Health Statistics*, series 23, no. 26 (May 2006).

[60] Jacqueline E. Darroch, David J. Landry, and Selene Oslak, "Age Differences Between Sexual Partners In the United States," *Family Planning Perspectives*, vol. 31, no. 4 (July/August 1999), Guttmacher Institute.

[61] Suzanne Ryan, Kerry Franzetta, Jennifer S. Manlove, and Erin Schelar, "Older Sexual Partners During Adolescence: Links to Reproductive Health Outcomes in Young Adulthood," *Perspectives on Sexual and Reproductive Health*, vol. 40, no. 1 (March 2008), Guttmacher Institute.

[62] David J. Landry and Jacqueline D. Forrest, "How Old Are U.S. Fathers?" *Family Planning Perspectives*, vol. 27, no. 4 (1995).

[63] Jacqueline E. Darroch, David J. Landry, and Selene Oslak, "Age Differences Between Sexual Partners In the United States," *Family Planning Perspectives*, vol. 31, no. 4 (July/August 1999), Guttmacher Institute.

[64] The following families automatically qualify for CSE services (free of charge): families receiving (or who formerly received) Temporary Assistance to Needy Families (TANF) benefits (Title IV-A of the Social Security Act), foster care payments, or Medicaid coverage. Other families must apply for CSE services, and states must charge an application fee that cannot exceed $25. In FY2006, the CSE caseload consisted of 15.8 million cases, of

which 2.3 million were TANF cases; 7.3 million were former-TANF cases, and 6.2 million had never been on TANF.

[65] These 10.4 million children who were born outside of marriage represented about 60% of the children in the CSE caseload in 2006.

[66] Office of Child Support Enforcement (HHS), "Child Support Enforcement, FY 2006 (preliminary report)," March 2007.

[67] Among custodial parents (living with children under age 21) who actually received child support payments in 2005 (latest available data), 41% were divorced, 25% were married, 24% were never married, 9% were separated, and 1% were widowed. Source: U.S. Census Bureau, "Custodial Mothers and Fathers and Their Children: 2005," *Current Population Reports*, P60-234 (August 2007), Table 4.

[68] Laurene T. McKillop with preface by Judith Cassetty, "Benefits of Establishing Paternity," U.S. Department of Health and Human Services, Office of Child Support Enforcement, (June 1981, reprinted September 1985), p. ix-xii.

[69] For an array of information on the impact of father involvement in their children's lives, see the following website: National Child Care Information and Technical Assistance Center (HHS), "Father Involvement in Children's Development," [http://nccic.acf.hhs.gov/poptopics/fatherinvolvement.html].

[70] Dore Hollander, "Nonmarital Childbearing in the United States: A Government Report," *Family Planning Perspectives*, vol. 28, no. 1 (January-February 1996), p. 31.

[71] Kathryn Edin and Maria Kefalas, "Promises I Can Keep: Why Poor Women Put Motherhood Before Marriage," University of California Press, 2005, p. 136.

[72] In general, the use of contraceptives has increased substantially over the last twenty years and women have become more proficient in properly using contraceptives. Thus, contraceptive misuse or non-use is not discussed in this report as a reason for increased nonmarital childbearing. Nonetheless, it is important to note that shifts in the types of contraceptives used has had offsetting influences on the risk of unintended pregnancy. The chances of contraceptive failure (including method failure and incorrect or inconsistent use) in the first 12 months of use are higher for the condom (14%) than for oral contraceptives (8%), and lowest for injectables (3%), implants (2%), and sterilization. Thus, the mix of methods used by women included greater proportions of both more effective and less effective methods. Source: Stephanie J. Ventura and Christine A. Bachrach, "National Vital Statistics Reports," vol. 48, no. 16, October 18, 2000, p. 9.

[73] Stephanie J. Ventura and Christine A. Bachrach, "Nonmarital Childbearing in the United States, 1940-99," Department of Health and Human Services, Centers for Disease Control and Prevention, National Center for Health Statistics, *National Vital Statistics Reports*, vol. 48, no. 16 (October 18, 2000), p. 3.

[74] Some analysts note that the economic returns associated with a college education are also a factor in marriage postponement. They contend that for many youth, college delays "adulthood" well into a person's twenties.

[75] Andrew J. Cherlin, "American Marriage in the Early Twenty-First Century," *The Future of Children*, vol. 15, no. 2 (Fall 2005).

[76] Ibid.

[77] Steven L. Nock, "Marriage as a Public Issue," *The Future of Children*, vol. 15, no. 2 (Fall 2005).

[78] Andrew J. Cherlin, "American Marriage in the Early Twenty-First Century," *The Future of Children*, vol. 15, no. 2 (Fall 2005). Also see Barbara Dafoe Whitehead, "Dan Quayle Was Right," *The Atlantic* (April 1993).

[79] Barbara Dafoe Whitehead and David Popenoe, "Changes in Teen Attitudes Toward Marriage, Cohabitation and Children: 1975-1995," 1999.

[80] Steven L. Nock, "Marriage as a Public Issue," *The Future of Children*, vol. 15, no. 2 (Fall 2005).

[81] Daniel T. Lichter, George Kephart, Diane K. McLaughlin, and David J. Landry, "Race and the Retreat from Marriage: A Shortage of Marriageable Men?," *American Sociological Review*, vol. 57 (December 1992), p. 781-799.

[82] Dennis A. Ahlburg and Carol J. DeVita, "New Realities of the American Family," *Population Bulletin*, vol. 47, no. 2 (August 1992), p. 14. See also Scott J. South, "Sociodemographic Differentials in Mate Selection Preferences," *Journal of Marriage and the Family*, vol. 53, no. 4 (November 1991). p. 928-940.

[83] William Julius Wilson, "The Truly Disadvantaged: The Inner City, the Underclass, and Public Policy," The University of Chicago Press, 1987.

[84] Andrea Kane and Daniel T. Lichter, "Reducing Unwed Childbearing: The Missing Link in Efforts to Promote Marriage," *Center on Children and Families*, Brief no. 37 (April 2006).

[85] Dore Hollander, "Nonmarital Childbearing in the United States: A Government Report," *Family Planning Perspectives*, vol. 28, no. 1 (January-February 1996), p. 31.

[86] Marcia Carlson, Sara McLanahan, and Paula England, "Union Formation and Dissolution in Fragile Families," Fragile Families Research, Center for Research on Child Wellbeing, Princeton University, August 2002, p. 21.

[87] Paul R. Amato, "The Impact of Family Formation Change on the Well-Being of the Next Generation," *The Future of Children*, vol. 15, no. 2 (Fall 2005), p. 79.

[88] Lawrence L. Wu, "Cohort Estimates of Nonmarital Fertility for U.S. Women," February 2008.

[89] U.S. Census Bureau. Survey of Income and Program Participation (SIPP), 2004 Panel. 2007; [http://www.census.gov/population/www/socdemo/marr-div.html].

[90] Contrary to the public perception that premarital sex is much more common now than in the past, the study found that even among women who were born in the 1940s, nearly 90% had sex before marriage. Source: Guttmacher Institute, "Premarital Sex is Nearly Universal Among Americans, and Has Been for Decades," News Release (December 19, 2006).

[91] William D. Mosher, Anjani Chandra, and Jo Jones, "Sexual Behavior and Selected Health Measures: Men and Women 15-44 Years of Age, United States, 2002," National Center for Health Statistics, Advance Data from *Vital and Health Statistics*, no. 362 (September 15, 2005).

[92] Lawrence B. Finer, "Trends in Premarital Sex in the United States, 1954-2003," *Guttmacher Institute*, Public Health Reports, January-February 2007, vol. 122. See also *Guttmacher Institute* News Release, "Premarital Sex Is Nearly Universal Among Americans, and Has Been For Decades," (December 19, 2006).

[93] Douglas Kirby, "Emerging Answers: 2007 — Research Findings on Programs to Reduce Teen Pregnancy and Sexually Transmitted Diseases," The National Campaign to Prevent Teen and Unplanned Pregnancy, November 2007, p. 53-71. Note: Although there is a widely held perception that low self-esteem is a risk factor for teenage pregnancy, the empirical research does not reach such an unequivocal conclusion.

[94] Ibid., p. 69.

[95] Alan Guttmacher Institute, "Abortion in the United States: Incidence and Access to Services, 2005," *Perspectives of Sexual and Reproductive Health*, vol. 40, no. 1 (March 2008). See also Stephanie J. Ventura, Joyce C. Abma, William D. Mosher, and Stanley K. Henshaw, "Estimated Pregnancy Rates by Outcome for the United States, 1990-2004," *National Vital Statistics Reports*, vol. 56, no. 15 (April 14, 2008).

[96] U.S. Census Bureau, *Statistical Abstract of the United States: 2008*, Table 97.

[97] Note: The data in the text above is highlighting 2006 data related to living arrangements of children because the 2007 birth data is not yet available. The 2007 data related to living arrangements of children specifically includes a category titled " children living with both parents not married to each other" (i.e., cohabiting parents). In 2007, 67.8% of the 73.7 million U.S. children (under age 18) lived with both of their married parents, 2.9% lived with both parents who were not married, 17.9% lived with their mother, and 2.6% lived with their father. The other 8.8% of children lived with neither parent (3.5%) or lived with their mother (4.7%) or father (0.6%) who was separated (by absence or a "formal"

separation agreement) from the other parent. In general, if a woman has a child while she is formally married, the child's father is considered to be the woman's husband (regardless of whether or not he is "absent"). Note: In 2007, about 13% of the children living with their unmarried mothers ("mother-only families") were in a household that included non-relatives. A non-relative could be a stepfather, adoptive father, or the mother's significant other or it could be someone not romantically involved with the mother (e.g., a friend, male or female). U.S. Census Bureau, "America's Families and Living Arrangements: 2007," Table C3.

[98] Ariel Halpern and Elaine Sorensen, "Children's Environment and Behavior — Children Born Outside of Marriage," Snapshots of America's Families, Urban Institute, January 1, 1999.

[99] Although the early research did not distinguish between married and cohabiting parents, later research has found that cohabiting relationships are less stable than marriages and thereby from the standpoint of the child less desirable than marriages.

[100] Sara McLanahan and Gary Sandefur, Growing Up With a Single Parent: What Hurts, What Helps (Cambridge, MA: Harvard University Press, 1994); see also L. Bumpass, "Children and Marital Disruption: A Replication and Update," Demography, vol. 21(1984), pp. 71-82; see also Rebecca A. Maynard, ed., "Kids Having Kids: A Robin Hood Foundation Special Report on the Costs of Adolescent Childbearing" (New York, 1996); see also Mary Parke, "Are Married Parents Really Better for Children? What Research Says About the Effects of Family Structure on Child Well-Being," Center on Law and Social Policy, May 2003; see also Glenn Stanton, "Why Marriage Matters for Children," Focus on the Family, 1997.

[101] Barbara Dafoe Whitehead, "Dan Quayle Was Right," The Atlantic (April 1993).

[102] Current Population Survey, A joint effort between the Bureau of Labor Statistics and the Census Bureau. Annual Social and Economic (ASEC) Supplement. Table POVO5.

[103] David Popenoe, "The Controversial Truth: Two Parent Families Are Better," New York Times (December 26, 1992), p. A21.

[104] Mary Parke, Are Married Parents Really Better for Children? What Research Says About the Effects of Family Structure on Child Well-Being, Center on Law and Social Policy, May 2003.

[105] Benjamin Scafidi, "The Taxpayer Costs of Divorce and Unwed Childbearing: First-Ever Estimates for the Nation and for All Fifty States," Institute for American Values, Georgia Family Council, Institute for Marriage and Public Policy, and Families Northwest, April 2008.

[106] The report does not separately estimate the economic costs associated with nonmarital childbearing.

[107] Benjamin Scafidi, "The Taxpayer Costs of Divorce and Unwed Childbearing: First-Ever Estimates for the Nation and for All Fifty States," Institute for American Values, Georgia Family Council, Institute for Marriage and Public Policy, and Families Northwest, April 2008.

[108] Paul R. Amato and Rebecca A. Maynard, "Decreasing Nonmarital Births and Strengthening Marriage to Reduce Poverty," The Future of Children, vol. 17, no. 2 (Fall 2007), p. 130.

[109] The 3.6 million figure was derived by applying the 29% reduction rate to the 12.8 million children who were in families with below poverty-level income in 2007. Note: According to the Census Bureau, in 2007, 12.8 million of the nearly 73 million related children (under age 18) living in families were in families with poverty-level income. Also, in 1970, 85.2% of children lived with both parents; in 1980, 76.7%; in 1990, 72.5%; in 2000, 69.1%; and in 2007, 67.8%.

[110] Saul D. Hoffman, "By the Numbers: The Public Cost of Teen Childbearing," The National Campaign to Prevent Teen Pregnancy, October 2006.

[111] The report differentiates teens ages 17 and younger who give birth and those who are ages 18 through 19 who give birth and finds that $8.6 billion of the costs are associated with the younger teens and only $0.4 billion with the older teens.

[112] According to the report, the steady decline in the teen birth rate between 1991 and 2004 yielding costs savings of $3.6 billion ($2.0 billion from the TANF program, $1.4 billion from the Food Stamps program, and $0.2 billion from the housing programs).

[113] Saul D. Hoffman, "By the Numbers: The Public Cost of Teen Childbearing," *The National Campaign to Prevent Teen Pregnancy*, October 2006.

[114] Rob Stein, "U.S. Fertility Rate Hits 35-Year High, Stabilizing Population," *The Washington Post* (December 21, 2007), p. A11.

[115] James R. Wetzel, "American Families: 75 Years of Change," *Monthly Labor Review* (March 1990).

[116] Jane Lawler Dye, "Fertility of American Women: 2006," U.S. Census Bureau, *Current Population Reports*, P20-558 (August 2008).

[117] Because the number of persons immigrating to the U.S. continues to increase, the U.S. population would have continued to grow even though the U.S. was below the demographic replacement level of 2.1 births per woman.

[118] Lawrence L. Wu, "Cohort Estimates of Nonmarital Fertility for U.S. Women," February 2008.

[119] With respect to black women, this means that if unmarried women had not been having babies, the growth of the black population would have severely shrunk.

[120] Lawrence L. Wu, "Cohort Estimates of Nonmarital Fertility for U.S. Women," February 2008.

[121] U.S. Census Bureau News, CB08-123, "An Older and More Diverse Nation by Midcentury," August 14, 2008.

[122] Ibid.

[123] Ibid.

[124] Peter S. Bearman and Hannah Bruckner, "Promising the Future: Virginity Pledges as They Affect the Transition to First Intercourse," *American Journal of Sociology*, January 2001.

[125] Those opposed to the abstinence-only education approach generally favor a comprehensive sex education approach (discussed later), but also claim that abstinence-only programs often use medically inaccurate information regarding STDs, condoms, and other contraceptive devices. The Department of Health and Human Services (HHS) now requires grantees of abstinence education programs to sign written assurances in grant applications that the material and data they use are medically accurate.

[126] For more information on these abstinence education programs, see CRS Report RS20873, *Reducing Teen Pregnancy: Adolescent Family Life and Abstinence Education Programs*, by Carmen Solomon-Fears.

[127] Abstinence education funding totaled $79 million in FY2001, $100 million in FY2002, $115 million in FY2003, $135 million in FY2004, $168 million in FY2005, and $177 million in FY2006 and FY2007.

[128] The predecessor of the AFL program was the Adolescent Pregnancy program, which was enacted in 1978 (P.L. 95-626). The Adolescent Pregnancy program was designed to alleviate the negative consequences of pregnancy for the adolescent parent and her child. The Adolescent Pregnancy program was consolidated into the Maternal and Child Health Block Grant when the AFL program was enacted.

[129] States use a variety of methods to meet the federal matching requirement, such as state funds, private or foundation funds, matching funds from community-based grantees, and in-kind services (e.g., volunteer staffing and public service announcements).

[130] The CBAE program was known as the Special Projects for Regional and National Significance (SPRANS) until FY2005.

[131] Christopher Trenholm, Barbara Devaney, Ken Fortson, Lisa Quay, Justin Wheeler, and Melissa Clark, "Impacts of Four Title V, Section 510 Abstinence Education Programs (final report)," *Mathematica Policy Research, Inc.*, April 2007; [http://aspe.hhs.gov/hsp/abstinence07/].

[132] U.S. Department of Health and Human Services (HHS), "Report Released on Four Title V Abstinence Education Programs," HHS Press Office, April 13, 2007, [http://aspe.hhs.gov/hsp/abstinence07/factsheet.shtml].

133 Some contend that the abstinence-only approach leads to a substitution of other risky behaviors such as oral sex. They cite recent data that indicates that about 25% of virgin teens (15-19) have engaged in oral sex. Source: *Child Trends Data Bank. New Indicator on Oral Sex*, September 15, 2005, at [http://www.childtrendsdatabank.org/whatsNew.cfm].

134 For more information on sexual activity of high school students, see CRS Report RS20873, *Reducing Teen Pregnancy: Adolescent Family Life and Abstinence Education Programs*, by Carmen Solomon-Fears.

135 Peter S. Bearman and Hannah Bruckner, "Promising the Future: Virginity Pledges as They Affect the Transition to First Intercourse," *American Journal of Sociology*, January 2001.

136 This report uses the term sexually transmitted diseases (STDs) rather than sexually transmitted infections (STIs). In the literature the terms are often used interchangeably.

137 The Centers for Disease Control and Prevention (CDC) estimates that approximately 19 million new infections occur each year, almost half of them among young people ages 15 to 24. Source: "Trends in Reportable Sexually Transmitted Disease in the United States, 2006," November 13, 2007.

138 U.S. General Accounting Office, "Teen Pregnancy: State and Federal Efforts to Implement Prevention Programs and Measure Their Effectiveness, GAO/HEHS-99-4, November 1998.

139 The National Campaign to Prevent Teen Pregnancy, "Putting What Works To Work: Curriculum-Based Programs That Prevent Teen Pregnancy," 2007.

140 The report only examined studies that had been published in 2000 or later.

141 The National Campaign to Prevent Teen Pregnancy, "Putting What Works To Work: Curriculum-Based Programs That Prevent Teen Pregnancy," 2007. Note: There also are many reasons why programs are not considered successful. For example, in some cases the evaluation studies are limited by methodological problems or constraints because the approach taken is so multilayered that researchers have had difficulty disentangling the effects of multiple components of a program. In other cases, the approach may have worked for boys but not for girls, or vice versa. In some cases, the programs are very small, and thereby it is harder to obtain significant results. In other cases, different personnel may affect the outcomes of similar programs.

142 Bill Albert, "With One Voice 2007 — America's Adults and Teens Sound Off About Teen Pregnancy,"February 2007, p. 2; [http://www.teenpregnancy.org/resources/data/pdf/WOV2007_fulltext.pdf]

143 There appears to be significant public support for the involvement of religious groups in preventing teen pregnancy. When asked what organizations could do the best job of providing teen pregnancy prevention services, 39% said religious groups, 42% said nonreligious community groups, and 12% said government. (Source: The National Campaign to Prevent Teen Pregnancy, *Keeping the Faith: The Role of Religion and Faith Communities in Preventing Teen Pregnancy*, by Barbara Dafoe Whitehead, Brian L. Wilcox, and Sharon Scales Rostosky. September 2001.)

144 Jennifer Manlove, Angela Romano Papillio, and Erum Ikramullah, "Not Yet: Program To Delay First Sex Among Teens," The National Campaign to Prevent Teen Pregnancy and Child Trends, September 2004, p. 4.

145 Erin Schelar, Kerry Franzetta, and Jennifer Manlove, "Repeat Teen Childbearing: Differnces Across States and by Race and Ethnicity," *Child Trends*, Research Brief no. 2007-23, October 2007.

146 Kristin A. Moore, "Nonmarital Childbearing in the United States," Child Trends, Inc. in U.S. Department of Health and Human Services, National Center for Health Statistics, "Report to Congress on Out-of-Wedlock Childbearing," Executive Summary, September 1995 [DHHS pub. no. (PHS) 95-1257-1], p. 27.

147 As originally enacted and continuing under the Deficit Reduction Act, TANF law allows states to use block grant and Maintenance of Effort (MOE) funds for activities to further any TANF purpose, including promotion of the formation and maintenance of two-parent families. However, state expenditures in this category have generally been small.

[148] Public policy frequently financially punishes married couples. The U.S. tax code, for example, contains a marriage penalty for high-earner, two-income couples. The earned income tax credit penalizes lower-wage married couples. Moreover, welfare rules have frequently made it harder for married households than for single-parent households to get benefits. Source: Wade F. Horn, "Wedding Bell Blues: Marriage and Welfare Reform," The Brookings Institute, Summer 2001.

[149] CRS Report RS22369, *TANF, Child Care, Marriage Promotion, and Responsible Fatherhood Provisions in the Deficit Reduction Act of 2005 (P.L. 109-171)*, by Gene Falk. March 1, 2007. Also see Healthy Marriage Initiative Home Page, [http://www.acf.hhs.gov/healthymarriage/index.html]

[150] Anne Menard and Oliver Williams, *It's Not Healthy If It's Not Safe: Responding to Domestic Violence Issues Within Healthy Marriage Programs*, November 2005 (updated May 2006), p. 2.

[151] Kathryn Edin and Maria Kefalas, "Promises I Can Keep: Why Poor Women Put Motherhood Before Marriage," University of California Press, 2005.

[152] U.S. Government Accountability Office, "Healthy Marriage and Responsible Fatherhood Initiative — Further Progress Is Needed in Developing a Risk-Based Monitoring Approach to Help HHS Improve Program Oversight," GAO-08-1002, September 2008.

[153] U.S. Congress, House Ways and Means Subcommittee on Human Resources, "Hearing On Fatherhood Legislation," Statement of Chairman Nancy Johnson. 106th Congress, 1st Session (October 5, 1999), p. 4.

[154] CRS Report RL31025, *Fatherhood Initiatives: Connecting Fathers to Their Children*, by Carmen Solomon-Fears. Also see Promoting Responsible Fatherhood Home Page, [http://fatherhood.hhs.gov/index.shtml].

[155] Information on the responsible fatherhood grants in each of the 10 HHS regions is available at [http://www.acf.hhs.gov/programs/ofa/hmabstracts/index.htm].

[156] See Karin Martinson and Demetra Nightingale, "Ten Key Findings from Responsible Fatherhood Initiatives," *The Urban Institute*, February 2008.

[157] John M. Martinez and Cynthia Miller, "Working and Earning: The Impact of Parents' Fair Share on Low-Income Fathers' Employment" (New York: MDRC, October 2000). Also see Cynthia Miller and Virginia Knox, "The Challenge of Helping Low-Income Fathers Support Their Children: Final Lessons from Parents' Fair Share" (New York: MDRC, November 2001), pp. v-vi.

[158] Sara McLanahan, "Testimony before the Mayor's Task Force on Fatherhood Promotion, National Fatherhood Summit," Washington, D.C., June 14, 1999.

[159] Jessica Pearson, Nancy Thoennes, and Lanae Davis, with Jane Venohr, David Price, and Tracy Griffith, "OCSE Responsible Fatherhood Programs: Client Characteristics and Program Outcomes" (Washington: U.S. Department of Health and Human Services, Administration for Children and Families, Center for Policy Research and Policy Studies, September 2003).

[160] Ibid.

[161] U.S. Government Accountability Office, "Healthy Marriage and Responsible Fatherhood Initiative — Further Progress Is Needed in Developing a Risk-Based Monitoring Approach to Help HHS Improve Program Oversight," GAO-08-1002, September 2008.

[162] In 2006, 25% of Title X clients were ages 19 or younger. CRS Report RL33644, *Title X (Public Health Service Act) Family Planning Program*, by Angela Napili.

[163] Dore Hollander, "Nonmarital Childbearing in the United States: A Government Report," *Family Planning Perspectives*, vol. 28, No. 1 (January-February 1996), p. 31.

[164] Patrick F. Fagan, "Promoting Adoption Reform: Congress Can Give Children Another Chance," *The Heritage Foundation*, Backgrounder #1080, May 6, 1996.

[165] Ibid.

[166] National Council For Adoption, "Adoption Factbook IV," 2007, p. 5.

[167] Child Welfare Information Gateway, "How Many Children Were Adopted in 2000 and 2001?"(U.S. Department of Health and Human Services, Children's Bureau), August 2004, pp. 15-17.

[168] Ibid., p. 263.

[169] Child support is paid until the child is age 18 (the age limit is higher is some states). Past-due child support (i.e., child support arrearages) are still owed even though the child has reached age 18 — in some states for an additional five to seven years, in some states to age 30.

[170] Paula Roberts, "The Importance of Child Support Enforcement: What Recent Social Science Research Tell Us," *Center for Law and Social Policy*, Spring 2002, p. 5.

[171] Chien-Chung Huang, "The Impact of Child Support Enforcement on Nonmarital and Marital Births: Does It Differ by Racial and Age Groups?," Joint Center for Policy Research, November 20, 2001, pp. 5-6.

[172] Daniel T. Lichter, "Marriage as Public Policy," *Progressive Policy Institute*, Policy Report, September 2001.

[173] Although P.L. 104-193 seeks to reduce pregnancies, birth data, and not pregnancy data, have become the indicator because birth data are more current and reliable.

[174] U.S. Congress. House. Committee on Ways and Means. *Green Book:2008*, Section 7. 2008. pp. 7-92;[http://waysandmeans.house.gov/Documents.asp?section=2168].

[175] Paula Roberts, "Out of Order? Factors Influencing the Sequence of marriage and Childbirth Among Disadvantaged Americans, Center for Law and Social Policy, *Couples and Marriage Series*, Brief no. 9 (January 2007).

[176] Barbara Dafoe Whitehead, "Dan Quayle Was Right," *The Atlantic* (April 1993).

[177] Andrew J. Cherlin, "American Marriage in the Early Twenty-First Century," *The Future of Children*, vol. 15, no. 2 (Fall 2005). Also see Barbara Dafoe Whitehead, "Dan Quayle Was Right," *The Atlantic* (April 1993).

[178] Paula Roberts, "Out of Order? Factors Influencing the Sequence of marriage and Childbirth Among Disadvantaged Americans, Center for Law and Social Policy, *Couples and Marriage Series*, Brief no. 9 (January 2007).

[179] Barbara Dafoe Whitehead, "Dan Quayle Was Right," *The Atlantic* (April 1993).

[180] Linda C. McClain, "Love, Marriage, and the Baby Carriage: Revisiting the Channelling Function of Family Law," Hofstra Univ. Legal Studies Research Paper no. 07-14, April 2007.

[181] Theodora Ooms, "The Role of Government in Strengthening Marriage," Center for Law and Social Policy, *Virginia Journal of Social Policy & the Law*, vol. 9:1 (2001).

[182] This report does not discuss childbearing (biological child of one member of the couple, adoption or through new reproductive technologies, such as sperm donation, egg donation, or surrogate birth mothers) or childrearing with respect to gay couples. For a discussion of the subject, see William Meezan and Jonathan Rauch, "Gay Marriage, Same-Sex Parenting, and America's Children," *The Future of Children*, vol. 15, no. 2 (Fall 2005), p. 97-115.

[183] Laura Duberstein Lindberg and Susheela Singh, "Sexual Behavior of Single Adult American Women," *Perspectives on Sexual and Reproductive Health*, vol. 40, no. 1 (March 2008).

[184] Andrew J. Cherlin, "American Marriage in the Early Twenty-First Century," *The Future of Children*, vol. 15, no. 2 (Fall 2005) p. 33.

[185] Cassandra Logan, Jennifer Manlove, Erum Ikramullah, and Sarah Cottingham, "Men Who Father Children with More Than One Woman: A Contemporary Portrait of Multiple-Partner Fertility," *Child Trends*, Research Brief no. 2006-10 (November 2006).

[186] Christina M. Gibson-Davis and Katherine A. Magnuson, "Explaining the Patterns of Child Support Among Low-Income Non-Custodial Fathers," December 2005. Also see Ronald B. Mincy, "Who Should Marry Whom?: Multiple Partner Fertility Among New Parents," Columbia University, February 2002. See also Paula Roberts, "The Implications of Multiple Partner Fertility for Efforts to Promote Marriage in Programs Serving Low-Income Mothers and Fathers," *Center for Law and Social Policy*, Policy Brief no. 11 (March 2008).

[187] The healthy marriage program and the responsible fatherhood program are designed to accommodate individuals of all ages, although individual programs may cater to persons in specific age groups. Administrators of the programs point out that the message of the programs are applicable to persons of all ages, from teens to middle-aged couples.

[188] Although several evaluations are underway to scientifically determine whether healthy marriage programs and responsible fatherhood programs work, they are many years from impact findings. Most are still at the initial stage of providing information on the implementation of the programs.

[189] The animosity mainly centered around funding concerns — in some of the early proposals marriage promotion initiatives were earmarked up to five times as much money as fatherhood initiatives. Supporters of responsible fatherhood programs argued that the promotion of marriage debate was overshadowing the precept that fathers should participate in the lives of their children regardless of the marital status of the parents.

[190] Also, it is interesting to note that many analysts contend that the many of the "soft skills" individuals learn in healthy marriage or responsible fatherhood programs are transferrable to the workplace. They assert that skills such as being able to communicate effectively with others, being consistent, and being on-time are abilities that may help individuals gain entry into the workforce as well as help them advance in their jobs.

[191] Both abstinence-only education programs and comprehensive sex education programs are currently focused on middle-school and high-school aged children.

[192] Shari L. Dworkin and John Santelli, "Do Abstinence-Plus Interventions Reduce Sexual Risk Behavior among Youth?," Public Library of Science Medicine, September 18, 2007.

In: Nonmarital Childbearing: Trends,...   ISBN: 978-1-60741-756-9
Editor: Gilberto de la Rayes   © 2010 Nova Science Publishers, Inc.

Chapter 2

REDUCING TEEN PREGNANCY: ADOLESCENT FAMILY LIFE AND ABSTINENCE EDUCATION PROGRAMS*

Carmen Solomon-Fears
Specialist in Social Legislation
Domestic and Social Policy Division

SUMMARY

In 2007, 48% of students in grades 9-12 reported that they had experienced sexual intercourse; about 20% of female teens who have had sexual intercourse become pregnant each year. In recognition of the often negative, long-term consequences associated with teenage pregnancy, Congress has provided funding for the prevention of teenage and out-of-wedlock pregnancies. This report discusses three programs that exclusively attempt to reduce teenage pregnancy. The Adolescent Family Life (AFL) demonstration program was enacted in 1981 as Title XX of the Public Health Service Act, and the Abstinence Education program was enacted in 1996 as part of the welfare reform legislation. Also, since FY2001, additional funding

---

* This is an edited, reformatted and augmented version of a CRS Report for Congress publication dated July 2008.

for community-based abstinence education programs has been included in annual Department of Health and Human Services (HHS) appropriations. This report will be updated periodically.

INTRODUCTION

Since 1991, teen pregnancy, abortion, and birth rates have fallen considerably (after 14 years of decline, the teen birth rate increased from 40.5 per 1,000 females ages 15 to 19 in 2005 to 41.9 in 2006). In 2002 (latest available data), the pregnancy rate for teenagers was 75.4 per 1,000 females aged 15-19, down 35% from the 1991 level of 115.3. The 2002 teen pregnancy rate is the lowest recorded since 1973, when this series was initiated;[1] however, it still is higher than the teen pregnancy rates of most industrialized nations. According to a recent report on children and youth, in 2007, 33% of 9th graders reported having experienced sexual intercourse. The corresponding statistics for older teens were 44% for 10th graders, 56% for 11th graders, and 65% for 12th graders.[2] About 20% of female teens who have had sexual intercourse become pregnant each year.

For many years, there have been divergent views with regard to sex and young people. Many argue that sexual activity in and of itself is wrong if the persons are not married. Others agree that it is better for teenagers to abstain from sex but are primarily concerned about the negative consequences of sexual activity, namely unintended pregnancy and sexually transmitted diseases (STDs). These two viewpoints are reflected in two pregnancy prevention approaches. The Adolescent Family Life (AFL) program encompasses both views and provides funding for both prevention programs and programs that provide medical and social services to pregnant or parenting teens. The Abstinence Education program centers on the abstinence-only message and only funds programs that adhere solely to bolstering that message. (For information on Title X, which serves a much broader clientele than teens and pre-teens, see CRS Report RL33644, *The Title X Family Planning Program*, by Angela Napili.)

THE ADOLESCENT FAMILY LIFE PROGRAM

The AFL demonstration program was enacted in 1981 as Title XX of the Public Health Service Act (P.L. 97-35). It is administered by the Office of Adolescent Pregnancy Programs, Department of Health and Human Services (HHS). From 1981 until 1996, the AFL program was the only federal program that focused directly on the issues of adolescent sexuality, pregnancy, and parenting.[3]

Program Purpose

The AFL program was designed to promote — family involvement in the delivery of services, adolescent premarital sexual abstinence, adoption as an alternative to early parenting, parenting and child development education, and comprehensive health, education, and social services geared to help the mother have a healthy baby and improve subsequent life prospects for both mother and child.

Allowable Projects

The AFL program authorizes grants for three types of demonstrations: (1) projects provide "care" services only (i.e., health, education, and social services to pregnant adolescents, adolescent parents, their infant, families, and male partners); (2) projects which provide "prevention" services only (i.e., services to promote abstinence from premarital sexual relations for pre-teens, teens, and their families); and (3) projects which provide a combination of care and prevention services. Any public or private nonprofit organization or agency is eligible to apply for a demonstration grant. AFL projects can be funded for up to five years. Currently (2007-2008), the AFL program is supporting 67 demonstration projects across the country. (See [http://www.hhs.gov/opa/familylife/grantees/grantees.html].)

AFL care projects are required to provide comprehensive health, education, and social services (including life and career planning, job training, safe housing, decisionmaking and social skills), either directly or through partnerships with other community agencies, and to evaluate new approaches for implementing these services. AFL care projects are based within a variety of settings such as universities, hospitals, schools, public health departments, or community agencies. Many provide home visiting services and all have partnerships with diverse community agencies. Currently, 31 care projects are being funded. Since 1997, all AFL prevention projects that have been funded have been abstinence-only projects that were required to conform to the definition of abstinence education as defined in P.L. 104-193. Most of these projects try to reach students between the ages of 9 to 14 in public schools, community settings or family households; all involve significant interaction with parents to strengthen the abstinence message. Currently, 36 abstinence-only projects are being funded.[4]

Table 1. Adolescent Family Life Program
(appropriations in millions of dollars)

FY	Approp.	FY	Approp.	FY	Approp.	FY	Approp.
1982	11.080	1990	9.421	1998	16.709	2006	30.742
1983	13.518	1991	7.789	1999	17.700	2007	30.742
1984	14.918	1992	7.789	2000	19.327	2008	29.778
1985	14.716	1993	7.598	2001	24.377		
1986	14.689	1994	6.250	2002	28.900		
1987	14.000	1995	6.698	2003	30.922		
1988	9.626	1996	7.698	2004	30.720		
1989	9.529	1997	14.209	2005	30.742		

Evaluations and Research

Each demonstration project is required to include an internal evaluation component designed to test hypotheses specific to that project's service delivery model. The grantee contracts with an independent evaluator, usually one affiliated with a college or university in the grantee's state. The AFL program also authorizes funding of research grants dealing with various aspects of adolescent sexuality, pregnancy, and parenting. Research projects have examined factors that influence teenage sexual, contraceptive and fertility behaviors, the nature and effectiveness of care services for pregnant and parenting teens and why adoption is a little-used alternative among pregnant teenagers. Since 1982, the AFL program has funded 68 research projects.

ABSTINENCE EDUCATION

1996 Welfare Reform

P.L. 104-193, the 1996 welfare reform law, provided $250 million in federal funds specifically for the abstinence education program ($50 million per year for five years, FY1998-FY2002). Funds must be requested by states when they solicit Title V Maternal and Child Health (MCH) block grant funds and must be used exclusively for teaching abstinence. To receive federal funds, a state must match every $4 in federal funds with $3 in state funds.[5] This means that full funding for abstinence education must total at least $87.5 million annually. Although the Title V abstinence-only education block grant has not yet been reauthorized, the latest extension, contained in P.L. 110-275 (H.R. 6331), continues funding for the abstinence-only block grant through June 30, 2009. P.L. 105-33, enacted in 1997, included funding for a scientific evaluation of abstinence education programs; Mathematica Policy Research won the contract. (*See Impacts of Four Title V, Section 510 Abstinence Education Programs*, April 2007, at [http://www.mathematica.org/publications/PDFs/impactabstinence.pdf].)

To ensure that the abstinence-only message is not diluted, the law (P.L. 104-193, Section 510 of the Social Security Act) stipulated that the term "abstinence education" means an educational or motivational program that (1) has as its exclusive purpose, teaching the social, psychological, and health gains of abstaining from sexual activity; (2) teaches abstinence from sexual activity outside of marriage as the expected standard for all school-age children; (3) teaches that abstinence is the only certain way to avoid out-of-wedlock pregnancy, STDs, and associated health problems; (4) teaches that a mutually faithful monogamous relationship within marriage is the expected standard of human sexual activity; (5) teaches that sexual activity outside of marriage is likely to have harmful psychological and physical effects; (6) teaches that bearing children out-of-wedlock is likely to have harmful consequences for the child, the child's parents, and society; (7) teaches young people how to reject sexual advances and how alcohol and drug use increases vulnerability to sexual advances; and (8) teaches the importance of attaining self-sufficiency before engaging in sex.

WHAT IS ABSTINENCE?

It is becoming clear that parents, teachers, and teenagers are not in agreement on what constitutes abstinence. Teens are more likely than adults to believe that behaviors that cannot result in pregnancy constitute abstinence. Because pregnancy prevention together with avoidance of STDs are dual goals of the abstinence education program, some observers contend that it is time for programs to explicitly define what constitutes sexual activity. Others contend that specifying behaviors other than sexual intercourse violates a child's innocence and may provide ideas for experimentation.

Source: Lisa Remez, "Oral Sex among Adolescents: Is It Sex or Is It Abstinence?" *Family Planning Perspectives* (Alan Guttmacher Institute), 32(6), Nov-Dec. 2000, pp. 298-304.

In FY2007, all but 10 states (California, Connecticut, Maine, Minnesota, Montana, New Jersey, Pennsylvania, Rhode Island, Vermont, and Wyoming) and several territories sponsored an abstinence education program. Abstinence education programs launch media campaigns to influence attitudes and behavior, develop abstinence education curricula, revamp sexual education classes, and implement other activities focused on abstinence education. State funding is based on the proportion of low-income children in the state as compared to the national total. In FY2007, federal abstinence education funding ranged from $88,501 in Alaska to $4,777,916 in Texas.

Appropriations History

P.L. 106-246 appropriated $20 million for FY2001 to HHS under the Special Projects of Regional and National Significance (SPRANS) program for abstinence-only education for adolescents aged 12 through 18. P.L. 106-554 provided $30 million for FY2002 for the SPRANS abstinence education program; P.L. 107-116 increased SPRANS program funding from $30 million to $40 million for FY2002. The SPRANS program funding was increased by P.L. 108-7 to $55 million for FY2003, and byP.L.108-199 to $70 million for FY2004. P.L. 108-447 increased funding for the SPRANS program, now the Community-Based Abstinence Education (CBAE) program, to $100 million for FY2005. P.L. 109-149 increased funding for CBAE to $109 million for FY2006. P.L. 110-5 maintained funding for CBAE at $109 million for FY2007. P.L. 110-161 maintained funding for CBAE at $109 million for FY2008.

ISSUES

Comparable Funding for Abstinence Education

President Bush has indicated his support for abstinence education. As governor of Texas, he stated: "For children to realize their dreams, they must learn the value of abstinence. We must send them the message that of the many decisions they will make in their lives, choosing to avoid early sex is one of the most important. We must stress that abstinence isn't just about saying no to sex; it's about saying yes to a happier, healthier future."[6] The proposal he supported during his presidential campaign would have provided at least as much funding for abstinence education as was provided for teen contraception services under the Medicaid, family planning (Title X), and AFL programs, namely about $135 million annually.[7] As many as 27 other federal programs have a teen contraception component, but expenditures solely for this component could not be isolated.[8] For FY2008, abstinence education funding totals $177 million: $50 million for the abstinence block grant to states; $13 million for the AFL abstinence education projects; $109 million for the CBAE program (up to $10 million of which may be used for a national abstinence education campaign); and $4.5 million for an evaluation of the program.[9]

Abstinence-Only Versus Comprehensive Sexuality Education

According to a 1997 survey, among the 69% of public school districts that had a district-wide policy to teach sex education, 14% had a comprehensive policy that treated abstinence as one option for adolescents in a broader sexuality education program; 51% taught abstinence as the preferred option for teenagers, but also permitted discussion about contraception as an effective means of protecting against unintended pregnancy and disease (an abstinence-plus policy); and 35% taught abstinence as the only option outside of marriage, with discussion of contraception prohibited entirely or permitted only to emphasize its shortcomings (abstinence-only policy).[10]

Advocates of the abstinence education approach argue that teenagers need to hear a single, unambiguous message that sex outside of marriage is wrong and harmful to their physical and emotional health. They contend that youth can and should be empowered to say no to sex. They argue that supporting both abstinence and birth control is hypocritical and undermines the strength of an abstinence-only message. They also cite research that indicates that teens who take virginity pledges to refrain from sex until marriage appear to delay having sex longer than those teens who do not make such a commitment. (The study found that teens who publicly promise to postpone sex until marriage refrain from intercourse for about a year and a half longer than teens who did not make such a pledge.)[11] They argue that abstinence is the most effective means of preventing unwanted pregnancy and sexually transmitted diseases (including HIV/AIDS).

Advocates of the more comprehensive approach to sex education argue that today's youth need information and decision-making skills to make realistic, practical decisions about whether to engage in sexual activities. They contend that such an approach allows young people to make informed decisions regarding abstinence, gives them the information they need to set relationship limits and to resist peer pressure, and also provides them with information on the use of contraceptives and the prevention of sexually transmitted diseases.[12] They maintain that abstinence-only messages provide no protection against the risks of pregnancy and disease for those who are sexually active. They point out that teens who break their virginity pledges were less likely to use contraception the first time than teens who had never made such a promise.

The April 2007 Mathematica evaluation of the Title V Abstinence Education program found that program participants had just as many sexual partners as nonparticipants, had sex at the same median age as nonparticipants, and were just as likely to use contraception as nonparticipants. Supporters of the abstinence-only approach say that the evaluation only examined four programs and is thereby inconclusive. A recent compilation of experimentally designed evaluations of comprehensive sexual education programs found that some comprehensive programs that included contraception information, decision-making skills, and peer pressure strategies were successful in delaying sexual activity, improving contraceptive use, or preventing teen pregnancy.[13]

End Notes

[1] The Alan Guttmacher Institute, *U.S. Teenage Pregnancy Statistics: National and State Trends and Trends by Race and Ethnicity*, updated September 2006, p. 5.

[2] Centers for Disease Control and Prevention, *MMWR*, vol. 57, no. SS-4, *Youth Risk Behavior Surveillance — United States, 2007*, June 6, 2008, available at [http://www.cdc.gov/Healthy Youth/yrbs/pdf/yrbss07_mmwr.pdf].

[3] The predecessor of the AFL program was the Adolescent Pregnancy program, which was enacted in 1978 (P.L. 95-626). The Adolescent Pregnancy program was designed to alleviate the negative consequences of pregnancy for the adolescent parent and her child (i.e., the care component of the AFL program). The Adolescent Pregnancy program was consolidated into the Maternal and Child Health Block Grant when the AFL program was enacted.

[4] Abstinence-only education funding under the AFL program amounted to $9 million in FY2001, $10 million in each of the fiscal years FY2002-FY2004, and $13 million in each of the fiscal years FY2005-FY2008.

[5] States use a variety of methods to meet the federal matching requirement, such as state funds, private or foundation funds, matching funds from community-based grantees, and in-kind services (e.g., volunteer staffing, public service announcements, etc.).

[6] Campaign literature from georgebush.com, accessed by author on November 22, 2000.

[7] Some family planning experts caution that the spending data may be misleading because it includes much more than contraception services. They contend that family planning programs include a vast array of medical services beyond the prescription of a contraceptive method, including pap smears, breast exams, screening for STDs, and one-on-one counseling of teens.

[8] The MCH and Title XX social services block grants are among the HHS programs that provide contraceptive services to teens (GAO/HEHS-99-4, *Teen Pregnancy: State and Federal Efforts to Implement Prevention Programs and Measure Their Effectiveness*, November 1998). Also, Temporary Assistance for Needy Families (TANF) funds can be used for such services for teens.

[9] Abstinence funding: $79 million in FY2001, $100 million in FY2002, $115 million in FY2003, $135 million in FY2004, $168 million in FY2005, and $177 million in FY2006 and FY2007.

[10] David J. Landry, Lisa Kaeser, and Cory L. Richards, "Abstinence Promotion and the Provision of Information about Contraception in Public School Districts Sexuality Education Policies," *Family Planning Perspectives* (Guttmacher Institute), 31(6), November-December 1999, pp. 280 286.

[11] Peter S. Bearman and Hannah Bruckner, "Promising the Future: Virginity Pledges as They Affect the Transition to First Intercourse," *American Journal of Sociology*, January 2001.

[12] Some contend that the abstinence-only approach leads to a substitution of other risky behaviors such as oral sex. They cite recent data that indicates that about 25% of virgin teens (15-19) have engaged in oral sex. Source: *Child Trends Data Bank. New Indicator on Oral Sex*, September 15, 2005, at [http://www.childtrendsdatabank.org/whatsNew.cfm].

[13] The National Campaign to Prevent Teen Pregnancy, *Putting What Works To Work: Curriculum-Based Programs That Prevent Teen Pregnancy*, 2007.

In: Nonmarital Childbearing: Trends,...   ISBN: 978-1-60741-756-9
Editor: Gilberto de la Rayes   © 2010 Nova Science Publishers, Inc.

Chapter 3

TITLE X (PUBLIC HEALTH SERVICE ACT) FAMILY PLANNING PROGRAM*

Angela Napili
Information Research Specialist

SUMMARY

The federal government provides grants for voluntary family planning services through the Family Planning Program, Title X of the Public Health Service Act, codified at 42 U.S.C. § 300 to § 300a-6. The program, enacted in 1970, is the only domestic federal program devoted solely to family planning and related preventive health services. Title X is administered through the Office of Population Affairs (OPA) under the Office of Public Health and Science in the Department of Health and Human Services (DHHS). It receives its funding through appropriations for the Health Resources and Services Administration (HRSA) in DHHS.

Although the authorization for Title X ended with FY1985, funding for the program has continued to be provided through appropriations bills for the Departments of Labor, Health and Human Services, and Education, and

---

* This is an edited, reformatted and augmented version of a CRS Report for Congress publication dated January 2009.

Related Agencies (Labor-HHS-Education). The Title X program received $300 million for FY2008, 6% more than the FY2007 level of $283.1 million.

On September 30, 2008, President Bush signed P.L. 110-329, the Consolidated Security, Disaster Assistance, and Continuing Appropriations Act, 2009. P.L. 110-329 provides temporary FY2009 funding, at the FY2008 funding level, through March 6, 2009.

The law (42 U.S.C. § 300a-6) prohibits the use of Title X funds in programs where abortion is a method of family planning. According to OPA, family planning projects that receive Title X funds are closely monitored to ensure that federal funds are used appropriately and that funds are not used for prohibited activities such as abortion. The prohibition on abortion does not apply to all the activities of a Title X grantee, but only to activities that are part of the Title X project. A grantee's abortion activities must be "separate and distinct" from the Title X project activities.

Several bills addressing Title X have been introduced in the 111th Congress. The Prevention First Act (S. 21/H.R. 463) would authorize Title X appropriations of $700 million for FY2010 and "such sums as may be necessary for each subsequent fiscal year." Other introduced bills include H.R. 221, which would require assurances that family planning projects will provide pamphlets with adoption centers' contact information, and S. 85, which would prohibit Title X grants to abortion-performing entities.

In the December 19, 2008 *Federal Register,* DHHS published a rule that is intended to increase awareness of existing statutes that "protect the rights of health care entities/entities, both individuals and institutions, to refuse to perform health care services and research services to which they may object for religious, moral, ethical, or other reasons." Some critics have argued that the rule could limit patients' access to contraception, and that it conflicts with the Title X requirement that grantees provide pregnant women, upon request, nondirective counseling and referrals on several options including abortion.

TITLE X PROGRAM ADMINISTRATION
AND COVERED SERVICES

Title X is administered through the Office of Population Affairs (OPA) under the Office of Public Health and Science in the Department of Health and Human Services (DHHS). It receives its funding through the appropriation for the Health Resources and Services Administration. OPA administers three types of project grants under Title X: family planning services;[1] family planning personnel training;[2] and family planning service delivery improvement research grants.[3]

Grants for family planning services fund family planning and related preventive health services, such as infertility services; natural family planning methods; services to adolescents; adolescent abstinence counseling; breast and cervical cancer screening and prevention; and sexually transmitted disease (STD) and HIV prevention education, counseling, testing, and referral.[4] Priority for the provision of these services is to be given to lower-income families; grantees may use a sliding fee schedule for determining client contributions for care, but grantees may not charge low-income persons for care. The services must be provided "without coercion and with respect for the privacy, dignity, social, and religious beliefs of the individuals being served."[5]

Grants for family planning personnel training are to be used to train staff and "to improve utilization and career development of paraprofessional and paramedical manpower in family planning services, particularly in rural areas."[6] Staff are trained through 10 regional general training programs, one national clinical training program, one national training center, and one national training program focused on improving Title X services for males.[7] The family planning service delivery improvement research grants are to be used to develop studies to improve the delivery of family planning services. These research grants target projects that enhance effectiveness and efficiency of the service delivery system.

Title X clinics provide confidential screening, counseling, and referral for treatment. In this regard, OPA has indicated that the program is committed to maintaining the integration of HIVprevention services in all family planning clinics.[8] OPA provides supplemental funding for grants to help Title X projects implement the Centers for Disease Control and Prevention's "Revised Recommendations for HIV Testing of Adults, Adolescents, and Pregnant Women in Health Care Settings."[9] OPA has also affirmed that Title X's HIV/AIDS education activities should incorporate the "ABC" message: "extramarital abstinence" (A); "be faithful in marriage or committed relationships" (B); and "correct and consistent condom use" (C).[10]

In 2006, Title X grantees reported that 5% of their clients were male.[11] Common services that family planning agencies offer to males include condom provision, STD counseling, contraceptive counseling, and STD treatment and testing.[12]

Ninety percent of Title X funds are used for clinical services.[13] At the start of FY2008, there were 88 Title X family planning services grantees. Such grantees included 43 state or local health departments, 6 territorial health departments, 10 Planned Parenthood affiliates, and 29 other nonprofit organizations, such as hospitals, community health centers, family planning councils and universities.[14] Title X grantees can provide family planning services directly or they can delegate Title X monies to other agencies to provide services. Although there are no matching requirements for grants, regulations specify that no clinics may be fully supported by Title X funds.[15] Title X provides services through more than 4,400 clinics nationwide.[16]

In 2007, Title X served 4.987 million clients, primarily low-income women and adolescents.[17] 92% of clients had incomes at or below 200% of the federal poverty level.[18] For many clients, Title X clinics are their only continuing source of health care.[19] In 2007, the latest year for which data is available, 64% of Title X clients were uninsured.[20]

More information on the Title X program, including regional contacts, can be found on the Internet at http://www.hhs.gov/opa/familyplanning/.

FUNDING

Although the program is administered by OPA, funding for Title X activities is provided through the Health Resources and Services Administration (HRSA) in DHHS. Authorization of appropriations expired at the end of FY1985, but the program has continued to be funded through appropriations bills for the Departments of Labor, Health and Human Services, and Education, and Related Agencies (Labor-HHS-Education).

FY2009 Funding Proposals

On September 30, 2008, President Bush signed P.L. 110-329, the Consolidated Security, Disaster Assistance, and Continuing Appropriations Act, 2009. It provides temporary FY2009 funding, at the FY2008 funding level, through March 6, 2009. Under the continuing resolution, funds are made available under the same authority and conditions provided during FY2008.

On July 8, 2008, the Senate Appropriations Committee reported its proposed bill for FY2009 Labor-HHS-Education appropriations (S. 3230; S.Rept. 110-410). It would have provided $300.0 million for Title X, the same as the FY2008 funding level and President Bush's Budget Request.[21] The bill repeated previous years' language requiring grantees to certify that they encourage "family participation" when minors decide to seek family planning services, and to certify that they counsel minors on how to resist attempted coercion into sexual activity. The bill also repeated a clarification that family planning providers are not exempt from state notification and reporting laws on child abuse, child molestation, sexual abuse, rape, or incest.[22] In S.Rept. 110-410, the Senate Appropriations Committee instructed that family planning funds be distributed to regional offices within 60 days of the appropriation bill's enactment. The report also stated the committee's intention that "the regional offices should retain the authority for the review, award and administration of family planning funds, in the same manner and timeframe as in fiscal year 2006." In addition, the committee intended that at least 90% of appropriated Title X funds, as well as any remaining year-end funds, should be spent on clinical services.

On February 4, 2008, President Bush submitted the FY2009 Budget, which requested $300.0 million for Title X, the same as the FY2008 funding level. The Budget Justification explained that the program would continue to seek ways "to increase efficiencies" in the face of increasing medical care prices, and to "increase competition" for funds, targeting areas that lack access to family planning services. The Budget Justification noted, "Rising costs of medical care will make it difficult to maintain service delivery at FY2008 levels." The Administration expected the proposed FY2009 level to fund services to 4.985 million clients and to avert 978,000 unintended pregnancies (compared with serving an expected 5.000 million clients and preventing an expected 981,000 unintended pregnancies in FY2008).[23]

FY2008 Appropriations

On December 26, 2007, President Bush signed the Consolidated Appropriations Act, 2008 (P.L. 110-161), which provided $300.0 million for Title X in FY2008, 6% more than the FY2007 level of $283.1 million.[24]

The FY2008 Consolidated Appropriations Act repeated previous years' language that Title X funds not be spent on abortions, that all pregnancy counseling be nondirective, and that funds not be spent on "any activity (including the publication or distribution of literature) that in any way tends to promote public support or opposition to any legislative proposal or candidate for public office."[25] The law also repeated language requiring grantees to certify that they encourage "family participation" when minors decide to seek family planning services, and to certify that they counsel minors on how to resist attempted coercion into sexual activity.[26] The law also repeated a clarification that family planning providers are not exempt from state notification and reporting laws on child abuse, child molestation, sexual abuse, rape, or incest.[27]

The FY2008 Consolidated Appropriations Act's Explanatory Statement stated that in implementing the act, agencies should be guided by language and instructions in H.Rept. 110-231 and S.Rept. 110-107.[28] In S.Rept. 110-107, the Senate Appropriations Committee instructed that family planning funds be distributed to regional offices within 60 days of the appropriation bill's enactment. The report also stated the committee's intention that "the regional offices should retain the authority for the review, award and administration of family planning funds, in the same manner and timeframe as in fiscal year 2006." In addition, the committee intended that at least 90% of appropriated Title X funds, as well as any remaining year-end funds, should be spent on clinical services.[29]

The FY2008 Labor-HHS-Education appropriations law (P.L. 110-161, Division G) contained a provider conscience clause, which does not explicitly mention Title X, but which conflicts with Title X regulations on abortion referrals, according to some critics. Sometimes referred to as the Weldon Amendment, the clause states that "None of the funds made available in this Act may be made available to a Federal agency or program, or to a State or local government, if such agency, program, or government subjects any institutional or individual health care entity to discrimination on the basis that the health care entity does not provide, pay for, provide coverage of, or refer for abortions."[30] The Weldon Amendment was originally adopted as part of the FY2005 Labor-HHS-Education appropriations law, and has been attached to each subsequent Labor-HHS-Education appropriations law.[31]

Some have argued that the Weldon Amendment conflicts with regulations that require Title X family planning services projects to give pregnant women the opportunity to receive information, counseling, and referral upon request for several options including "pregnancy termination."[32] The regulation states that if the woman requests such information and counseling, the project must give "neutral, factual information and nondirective counseling on each of the options, and referral upon request, except with respect to any option(s) about which the pregnant woman indicates she does not wish to receive such information and counseling."[33]

In the December 19, 2008 *Federal Register,* DHHS published a final rule to increase awareness of the Weldon Amendment and two other provider conscience statutes. In the rule's preamble, DHHS agreed with commenters that the provider conscience statutes are inconsistent with the Title X regulations, so that in certain situations, OPA would not enforce the Title X regulatory requirements on objecting grantees or applicants.[34] The rule is discussed further in "Provider Conscience Rule" below.

ABORTION AND TITLE X

The law prohibits the use of Title X funds in programs where abortion is a method of family planning.[35] On July 3, 2000, OPA released a final rule with respect to abortion services in family planning projects.[36] The rule updated and revised regulations that had been in effect since 1988.[37] The major revision revoked the "gag rule," which restricted family planning grantees from providing abortion-related information. The regulation at 42 C.F.R. § 59.5 had required, and continues to require, that abortion not be provided as a method of family planning. The July 3, 2000 rule amended the section to add the requirement that a project must give pregnant women the opportunity to receive information and counseling on each of the following options: prenatal care and delivery; infant care, foster care, or adoption; and pregnancy termination. If the woman requests such information and counseling, the project must give "neutral, factual information and nondirective counseling on each of the options, and referral upon request, except with respect to any option(s) about which the pregnant woman indicates she does not wish to receive such information and counseling."[38]

According to OPA, family planning projects that receive Title X funds are closely monitored to ensure that federal funds are used appropriately and that funds are not used for prohibited activities such as abortion. The prohibition on abortion does not apply to all the activities of a Title X grantee, but only to activities that are part of the Title X project. The grantee's abortion activities must be "separate and distinct" from the Title X project activities.[39] Safeguards to maintain this separation include (1) careful review of grant applications to ensure that the applicant understands the requirements and has the capacity to comply with all requirements; (2) independent financial audits to examine whether there is a system to account for program-funded activities and non-allowable program activities; (3) yearly comprehensive reviews of the grantees' financial status and budget report; and (4) periodic and comprehensive program reviews and site visits by OPA regional offices.

Table 1. Title X Family Planning Program Appropriations (in millions)

FY Appropriation	FY Appropriation	FY Appropriation
1971 $6.0	1984 $140.0	1997 $198.5
1972 $61.8	1985 $142.5	1998 $203.5
1973 $100.6	1986 $136.4	1999 $215.0
1974 $100.6	1987 $142.5	2000 $238.9
1975 $100.6	1988 $139.7	2001 $253.9
1976 $100.6	1989 $138.3	2002 $265.0
1977 $113.0	1990 $139.1	2003 $273.4
1978 $135.0	1991 $144.3	2004 $278.3
1979 $135.0	1992 $149.6	2005 $286.0
1980 $162.0	1993 $173.4	2006 $282.9
1981 $161.7	1994 $180.9	2007 $283.1
1982 $124.2	1995 $193.3	2008 $300.0
1983 $124.1	1996 $192.6	2009 a

Source: FY1971-FY2005: Department of Health and Human Services, Office of Population Affairs, *Funding History*, http://www.hhs.gov/opa/about/budget/; FY2006: Senate Appropriations Committee, S.Rept. 109-287 (p. 325); FY2007-FY2008: *Consolidated Appropriations Act, 2008 Committee Print of the House Committee on Appropriations on H.R. 2764/Public Law 110-161*, p. 1793, http://www.gpoaccess.gov/congress/house/appropriations/08conappro.html; FY2009: DHHS, HRSA, *Fiscal Year 2009 Justification of Estimates for Appropriations Committees*, p. 249; Senate Appropriations Committee, S.Rept. 110-410 (p. 59).
a. Continuing resolution P.L. 110-329, signed into law September 30, 2008, provides temporary funding at the FY2008 level through March 6, 2009. President Bush's FY2009 Budget requested $300.0 million for Title X. The Senate-reported Labor-HHS-Education bill (S. 3230; S.Rept. 110-410) would provide $300.0 million for Title X in FY2009.

It is unclear exactly how many Title X clinics also provide abortions through their non-Title X activities. In 2004, following appropriations conference report directions, DHHS surveyed its Title X grantees on whether their clinic sites also provided abortions with non-federal funds.[40] Grantees were informed that responses were voluntary and "without consequence, or threat of consequence, to non-responsiveness." The survey did not request any identifying information. DHHS mailed surveys to 86 grantees and received 46 responses. Of these, nine indicated that at least one of their clinic sites (17 clinic sites in all) also provided abortions with non-federal funds, and 34 indicated that none of their clinic sites provided abortions with non-federal funds; three responses had no numerical data or said the information was unknown.

Title X supporters argue that family planning reduces unintended pregnancies, thereby reducingabortion.[41] On the other hand, Title X critics argue that federal funds should be withheld from any organization that performs or promotes abortions, such as the Planned Parenthood Federation of America. These critics argue that if a family planning program is operated by an organization that also performs abortions, the implicit assumption and the message to clients is that abortion is a method of family planning.[42]

TEENAGE PREGNANCY AND TITLE X

In 2007, 25% of Title X clients were aged 19 or younger.[43] Critics argue that by funding Title X, the federal government is implicitly sanctioning nonmarital sexual activity among teens. These critics argue that a reduced teenage pregnancy rate could be achieved if family planning programs emphasized efforts to convince teens to delay sexual activity, rather than efforts to decrease the percentage of sexually active teens who become pregnant.[44] (See CRS Report RS20873, *Reducing Teen Pregnancy: Adolescent Family Life and Abstinence Education Programs*, by Carmen Solomon-Fears, for a broader discussion of teen pregnancy.)

The program's supporters, on the other hand, argue that the Title X program should be expanded to serve more people in order to reduce the rate of unintended pregnancies. According to DHHS, in 2007, Title X family planning services helped avert an estimated 242,480 unintended teen pregnancies.[45] Supporters of expanding family planning services argue that the United States has a higher teen pregnancy rate than some countries (such as Sweden) where a similar percentage of teens are sexually active, in part because U.S. teens use contraception less consistently.[46]

PLANNED PARENTHOOD AND TITLE X

In May 2003, the General Accounting Office (GAO; now named the Government Accountability Office) updated a report on federal funds provided to several nonprofit organizations and their affiliates involved in health-related activities during FY2001.[47] The report provided information on the Planned Parenthood Federation of America, the Population Council, the International Planned Parenthood Federation, the Alan Guttmacher Institute, Advocates for Youth, and the Sexuality Information and Education Council of the United States (SIECUS). Information was collected from each organization with respect to their expenditure of federal funds. Only Planned Parenthood and the Alan Guttmacher Institute reported spending Title X funds.

Planned Parenthood operates through a national office and 97 affiliates. Affiliates participating in Title X receive funds directly and indirectly from other Title X grantees, such as their state or local health departments. Planned Parenthood also operates nearly 880 local health centers.[48] The Alan Guttmacher Institute is an affiliate of the Planned Parenthood Federation and provides policy analysis and conducts research. According to the GAO report, in FY2001 Planned Parenthood spent $58.7 million of Title X funds, and the Alan Guttmacher Institute spent $315,320 of such funds; together this amounts to approximately 23% of Title X appropriations for that year.

LEGISLATION IN THE 111TH CONGRESS

Several bills on the Title X program have been introduced in the 111th Congress.

Reauthorization

S. 21/H.R. 463, the Prevention First Act, was introduced in the Senate January 6, 2009, and in the House January 13, 2009. These companion bills would authorize Title X appropriations of $700 million for FY2010 and "such sums as may be necessary for each subsequent fiscal year." S. 21 was referred to the Senate Committee on Health, Education, Labor, and Pensions. H.R. 463 was referred to the House Committees on Energy and Commerce, Ways and Means, and Education and Labor.

Adoption Promotion

H.R. 221, the Adoption Information Act, was introduced January 6, 2009. It would require the DHHS Secretary to annually prepare, update, and distribute to each Title X service grantee pamphlets listing contact information for all adoption centers in the state where services are provided. Title X service projects would be required to provide "assurances satisfactory to the Secretary" that they will (1) give the pamphlet to each family planning client at the time the person inquires about services, (2) orally inform the client that the pamphlet is from DHHS and has a comprehensive list of adoption centers in the state, and (3) give the client "an opportunity to read the pamphlet." H.R. 221 was referred to the House Committee on Energy and Commerce.

Abortion Restrictions

S. 85, the Title X Family Planning Act, was introduced January 6, 2009. It would prohibit Title X funds from going to entities that perform abortions or whose subgrantees perform abortions, except in certain physician-certified cases where the woman is "in danger of death unless an abortion is performed." This prohibition would not apply to hospitals, unless the hospital subgrants to a non-hospital entity that performs abortions. S. 85 would require Title X grant applicants to certify that they and their subgrantees adhere to the abortion prohibition. It would also require the DHHS to provide Congress with an annual list of Title X grantees that perform abortions; if an entity appears on the list, it would be ineligible for subsequent fiscal year Title X funds unless it certifies that it no longer performs abortions. S. 85 was referred to the Senate Committee on Health, Education, Labor, and Pensions.

H.R. 614, the Title X Abortion Provider Prohibition Act, was introduced January 21, 2009. The bill would prohibit Title X assistance to any entity unless it certifies that it will not perform, nor provide funds to any other entity that performs, an abortion during the period of assistance. The prohibition would not apply to hospitals, unless the hospital provides funds to a non-hospital entity that performs an abortion. The bill has exceptions for abortions performed in cases of rape, incest against a minor, or certain physician-certified cases where the woman is "in danger of death unless an abortion is performed." H.R. 614 would also require the DHHS Secretary to provide Congress an annual report listing, for each entity receiving a Title X grant: information on any abortions it performed, the date that it last certified that it would not perform abortions, and any other entities to which it makes available funds received through Title X grants. H.R. 614 was referred to the House Committee on Energy and Commerce.

PROVIDER CONSCIENCE RULE

In the December 19, 2008 *Federal Register,* DHHS published the final rule "Ensuring That Department of Health and Human Services Funds Do Not Support Coercive or Discriminatory Policies or Practices in Violation of Federal Law."[49] The rule's stated purpose is to provide for the implementation and enforcement of several conscience clause laws (including the Weldon Amendment) that "protect the rights of health care entities/entities, both individuals and institutions, to refuse to perform health care services and research services to which they may object for religious, moral, ethical, or other reasons."[50]

The rule states that entities carrying out DHHS health service programs shall not require individuals "to perform or assist in the performance of any part of a health service program or research activity funded by the Department if such service or activity would be contrary to his religious beliefs or moral convictions."[51] The rule defines *assist in the performance* as participating in any activity with a "reasonable connection" to the objectionable procedure or health service, including "counseling, referral, training, and other arrangements" for the procedure or health service.[52]

The rule prohibits recipients of HHS appropriations act funds from subjecting institutions or individuals to discrimination because they do not refer patients for abortions.[53] Also, the rule prohibits recipients of grants under the Public Health Service Act from discriminating against physicians or other health care professionals because they refused to assist in the performance of sterilization or abortion based on religious beliefs or moral convictions.[54]

Certain recipients and subrecipients of DHHS funds, including recipients and subrecipients of grants under the Public Health Service Act, are required to certify their compliance with the provider conscience rule.[55] The rule is effective as of January 20, 2009.[56]

Before publishing the final rule, DHHS solicited public comments.[57] Some commenters argued that the rule is inconsistent with the Title X requirement that grantees provide pregnant women, upon request, nondirective counseling and referrals on several options including abortion.[58] DHHS responded that the provider conscience requirement does indeed conflict with the Title X requirement, so that in certain situations, OPA would not enforce the Title X referral regulation:

> With regards to the Title X program, Commenters are correct that the current regulatory requirement that grantees must provide counseling and referrals for abortion upon request (42 C.F.R. 59.5(a)(5)) is inconsistent with the health care provider conscience protection statutory provisions and this regulation. The Office of Population Affairs, which administers the Title X program, is aware of this conflict with the statutory requirements and, as such, would not enforce this Title X regulatory requirement on objecting grantees or applicants.[59]

The final rule does not define the term *abortion*. Some commenters argued that by not defining abortion as excluding contraception, the rule could jeopardize Title X programs. DHHS responded that "questions over the nature of abortion and the ending of a life are highly controversial and strongly debated," and so declined to issue a formal definition. DHHS added that "nothing in this rule alters the obligation of federal Title X programs to deliver contraceptive services to clients in need as authorized by law and regulation."[60]

Some commenters argued that the rule could make it difficult for Title X clinics to screen job applicants to ensure that staff are willing to provide contraceptive services. DHHS responded that job applicants would be unlikely to apply for, or be best qualified for, jobs where they object to the majority of the work. DHHS explained further:

> To the extent a health care employer's adverse decision is based on an applicant's inability to perform the essential functions of a job, the decision would not typically constitute discrimination under the regulation even if the applicant had expressed an unwillingness to perform those functions on conscience grounds. However, an adverse decision predicated on an applicant's alleged "inability" could constitute unlawful discrimination if the employer's stated reasons are pretextual; for example, if the employer is using the definition of essential functions as a pretext for excluding applicants with certain religious beliefs or moral convictions.[61]

In response to comments that the rule would restrict patients' access to contraception, DHHS responded that "we have found no evidence that these regulations will create new barriers in accessing contraception unless those contraceptives are currently delivered over the religious or moral objections of the provider." [62]

More background about the rule is in CRS Report RL33467, *Abortion: Legislative Response*, by Jon O. Shimabukuro, and CRS Report RL34703, *The History and Effect of Abortion Conscience Clause Laws*, by Jon O. Shimabukuro.

SUMMARY OF TITLE X OF THE PUBLIC HEALTH SERVICE ACT

Below is a summary of Title X of the Public Health Service Act, codified at 42 U.S.C. § 300 to § 300a-6, Population Research and Voluntary Family Planning Programs:

Section 1001. Project Grants and Contracts for Family Planning Services

The Secretary may make grants to and enter into contracts with public or nonprofit private entities to assist in the establishment and operation of voluntary family planning projects to offer a broad range of acceptable and effective family planning methods and services (including natural family planning methods, infertility services, and services for adolescents). Entities which receive grants or contracts must encourage family participation in their projects.

Section 1002. Formula Grants to States for Family Planning Services

The Secretary may make grants to state health authorities to assist in planning, establishing, maintaining, coordinating, and evaluating family planning services. The state health authority must have an approved state plan for a coordinated and comprehensive program of family planning services.

Section 1003. Training Grants and Contracts

The Secretary may make grants to public or nonprofit private entities and enter into contracts with public or private entities and individuals to provide the training for personnel to carry out family planning service programs.

Section 1004. Research

The Secretary may conduct and make grants to public or nonprofit private entities and enter into contracts with public or private entities and individuals for projects for research in the biomedical, contraceptive development, behavioral, and program implementation fields related to family planning and population.

Section 1005. Informational and Educational Materials

The Secretary may make grants to public or nonprofit private entities and enter into contracts with public or private entities and individuals to assist in developing and making available family planning and population growth information (including educational materials) to all persons desiring such information.

Section 1006. Regulations and Payments

The Secretary may promulgate regulations and must determine the conditions for making payments to grantees to assure that such grants will be effectively utilized for the purposes they were made.

Grantees must assure that (1) priority will be given to the furnishing of services to persons from low-income families; and (2) no charge will be made in such project or program for services provided to any person from a low-income family except to the extent that payment will be made by a third party (including a government agency) which is authorized or is under legal obligation to pay the charge.

The Secretary must be satisfied that informational or educational materials developed or made available under the grant or contract will be suitable for the purposes of this title and for the population or community to which they are to be made available.

In the case of any grant or contract under Section 1001, such assurances shall provide for the review and approval of the suitability of such materials, prior to their distribution, by an advisory committee established by the grantee or contractor in accordance with regulations.

Section 1007. Voluntary Participation

The acceptance by any individual of family planning services or family planning or population growth information (including educational materials) shall be voluntary and shall not be a prerequisite to eligibility for or receipt of any other service or assistance from, or to participation in, any other program of the entity or individual that provided such service or information.

Section 1008. Prohibition of Abortion

None of the funds appropriated under this title shall be used in programs where abortion is a method of family planning.

AUTHOR CONTACT INFORMATION

Angela Napili
Information Research Specialist
anapili@crs.loc.gov, 7-0135

End Notes

[1] *Catalog of Federal Domestic Assistance (CFDA)*, Program number 93.217, http://www.cfda.gov.
[2] *CFDA*, Program number 93.260.
[3] *CFDA*, Program number 93.974.
[4] U.S. Department of Health and Human Services (DHHS), Office of Population Affairs, *Program Priorities*, http://www.hhs.gov/opa/familyplanning/policyplanningeval/

programpriorities/index.html.

[5] *CFDA*, Program number 93.217.

[6] *CFDA*, Program number 93.260.

[7] DHHS, Health Resources and Services Administration (HRSA), *Fiscal Year 2009 Justification of Estimates for Appropriations Committees*, p. 249,ftp://ftp.hrsa.gov/about/budgetjustification09.pdf.

[8] DHHS, Office of Population Affair (OPA), *HIV Prevention and Integration in Family Planning*, http://www.hhs.gov/opa/initiatives/hivprevention/

[9] Centers for Disease Control and Prevention (CDC), "Revised Recommendations for HIV Testing of Adults, Adolescents, and Pregnant Women in Health-Care Settings," *MMWR Recommendations and Reports*, vol. 55, no. RR-14 (September 26, 2006), pp. 1-17, http://www.cdc.gov/mmwr/preview/mmwrhtml/rr5514a1.htm. See also CDC, *HIV Testing in Healthcare Settings*, http://www.cdc.gov/hiv/topics/testing/healthcare/.

[10] DHHS, OPA, *Key Issues*, http://www.hhs.gov/opa/familyplanning/policyplanningeval/keyissues/keyissues.html.

[11] Christina Fowler, Julia Gable, and Jiantong Wang, *Family Planning Annual Report: 2007 National Summary*, RTI International, Research Triangle Park, NC, November 2008, pp. 9, 11, http://www.hhs.gov/opa/familyplanning/toolsdocs/fpar_2007_natl_summ.pdf.

[12] "Services for Men at Publicly Funded Family Planning Agencies, 1998-1999," *Perspectives on Sexual and Reproductive Health*, vol. 35, no. 5, September/October 2003. DHHS, OPA/Office of Family Planning, *FY 2003 Office of Family Planning Male Grantees Program Summaries*, http://www.hhs.gov/opa/familyplanning/grantees/maleinvolvement/.

[13] DHHS, HRSA, *Fiscal Year 2009 Justification of Estimates for Appropriations Committees*, pp. 249, 286.

[14] DHHS, HRSA, *Fiscal Year 2009 Justification of Estimates for Appropriations Committees*, p. 249. Email correspondence between the author and Maurice Huguley, Office of the Assistant Secretary for Legislation, U.S. Department of Health and Human Services, January 27, 2009.

[15] 42 C.F.R. § 59.7(c).

[16] DHHS, HRSA, *Fiscal Year 2009 Justification of Estimates for Appropriations Committees*, p. 249. A searchable directory of Title X providers is at OPA Clearinghouse, *Family Planning Database*, http://www.opaclearinghouse.org/db_search.asp.

[17] *Family Planning Annual Report: 2007 National Summary*, p. 8-9.

[18] *Family Planning Annual Report: 2007 National Summary*, p. 22.

[19] DHHS, HRSA, *Fiscal Year 2009 Justification of Estimates for Appropriations Committees*, pp. 249, 252.

[20] *Family Planning Annual Report: 2007 National Summary*, p. 21, 23.

[21] S.Rept. 110-410, p. 59.

[22] S. 3230 as placed on Senate Calendar, July 8, 2008, §§ 209-210.

[23] DHHS, HRSA, *Fiscal Year 2009 Justification of Estimates for Appropriations Committees*, pp. 249-252.

[24] This figure includes the act's across-the-board reduction of 1.747% for items in the Labor-HHS-Education division. The Consolidated Appropriations Act (P.L. 110-161) Division G, on Labor-HHS-Education appropriations, applies the reduction to accounts, items, programs, projects, and activities in the bill text and the Explanatory Statement narrative, with some exceptions (Title V, § 528).

[25] P.L. 110-161, Division G, Title II, 121 Stat. 2170.

[26] P.L. 110-161, Division G, Title II, sec. 210, 121 Stat. 2185. A recent evaluation of family involvement strategies found that "Barriers to parental participation are quite pronounced, with logistics, psychosocial factors, relationship dynamics and cultural issues among the obstacles." See RTI International, *An Assessment of Parent Involvement Strategies in Programs Serving Adolescents: Interim Report*, 2006, http://www.rti.org/pubs/assess

_parent.pdf; and DHHS, HRSA, *Fiscal Year 2009 Online Performance Appendix*, p. 156, ftp://ftp.hrsa.gov/about/performanceappendix09.pdf.

[27] P.L. 110-161, Division G, Title II, sec. 211. The DHHS Office of Inspector General recently reviewed OPA's activities to address state reporting requirements. It found that "OPA has informed and periodically reminds Title X grantees of their responsibilities" regarding these requirements, and that OPA addresses state reporting requirements in its site visits and reviews of grantees. See DHHS, Office of the Inspector General, *Federal Efforts to Address Applicable Child Abuse and Sexual Abuse Reporting Requirements for Title X Grantees*, Report no. OEI-02-03-00530, April 25, 2005, http://oig.hhs.gov/oei/reports/oei-02-03-00530.pdf.

[28] House Committee on Appropriations, *Consolidated Appropriations Act, 2008 Committee Print of the House Committee on Appropriations on H.R. 2764/Public Law 110-161*, pp. 1461-1462, http://www.gpoaccess.gov/congress/house/appropriations/08conappro.html.

[29] S.Rept. 110-107, pp.62-63.

[30] Consolidated Appropriations Act, 2008, P.L. 110-161, Division G, Departments Of Labor, Health And Human Services, and Education, and Related Agencies Appropriations Act, 2008, §508(d), 121 Stat. 1844.

[31] P.L. 108-447, Division F, §508(d), 118 Stat. 3163 (FY2005); P.L. 109-149, § 508(d), 119 Stat. 2879 (FY2006). Under P.L. 110-5, §2, 121 Stat. 8, FY2007 appropriations were subject to the same conditions as during FY2006. Under P.L. 110-329, Division A, §101, 122 Stat. 3574-3575, FY2009 continuing appropriations are subject to the same conditions as during FY2008.

[32] Examples of this argument appear in "Weldon Amendment," *Congressional Record*, daily edition, vol. 151, no. 51 (April 25, 2005), p. S4222; and "Federal Refusal Clause," *Congressional Record*, daily edition, vol. 151, no. 52 (April 26, 2005), p. S425. The National Family Planning and Reproductive Health Association (NFPRHA), many of whose members provide Title X services, filed a lawsuit challenging the Weldon Amendment in the U.S. District Court for the District of Columbia. The court found that "While Weldon may not provide the level of guidance that NFPRHA or its members would prefer, may create a conflict with pre-existing agency regulations, and may impose conditions that NFPRHA members find unacceptable, none of these reasons provides a sufficient basis for the court to invalidate an act of Congress in its entirety." Upon appeal, the U.S. Court of Appeals for the District of Columbia Circuit found that the plaintiff lacked the standing to challenge the Weldon Amendment. *See National Family Planning and Reproductive Health Association, Inc., v. Alberto Gonzales, et al.*, 468 F.3d 826 (D.C. Cir. 2006), and 391 F. Supp. 2d 200, 209 (D.D.C. 2005).

[33] 42 C.F.R. § 59(a)(5).

[34] 73 *Federal Register* 78087.

[35] 42 U.S.C. § 300a-6. In addition, so-called "Hyde amendments" to Departments of Labor, Health and Human Services, and Education, and Related Agencies Appropriations bills have also restricted federal abortion funding. For more background, see CRS Report RL33467, *Abortion: Legislative Response*, by Jon O. Shimabukuro.

[36] DHHS, OPA, "Standards of Compliance for Abortion-Related Services in Family Planning Services Projects," 65 *Federal Register* 41270–41280, July 3, 2000, and DHHS, OPA, "Provision of Abortion-Related Services in Family Planning Services Projects, " 65 *Federal Register* 41281-41282, July 3, 2000.

[37] 42 C.F.R. Part 59, "Grants for family planning services."

[38] On December 19, 2008, DHHS published a provider conscience rule which, according to DHHS, is inconsistent with the requirement that Title X grantees provide clients with abortion referrals upon request. 73 *Federal Register* 78087. This is also discussed below in "Provider Conscience Rule."

[39] 65 *Federal Register* 41281-41282, July 3, 2000.

[40] DHHS, *Report to Congress Regarding the Number of Family Planning Sites Funded Under Title X of the Public Health Service Act That Also Provide Abortions with Non-Federal Funds*, 2004. The DHHS was directed to conduct the survey by FY2004 appropriations conference report H.Rept. 108-401, pp. 800-801.

[41] An example of this argument can be found in U.S. Congress, Senate Committee on Appropriations, Subcommittee on Labor, Health and Human Services, and Education, *Threat to Title X and Other Women's Health Services*, 104th Cong., 1st sess., August 10, 1995, S.Hrg. 104-416 (Washington: GPO, 1996), pp. 16-21. See also Rachel Benson Gold, "Title X: Three Decades of Accomplishment," *The Guttmacher Report on Public Policy*, vol. 4, no. 1 (February 2000), p. 7. According to DHHS, in FY2006, Title X family planning services helped avert 975,080 unintended pregnancies (DHHS, HRSA, *Fiscal Year 2009 Justification of Estimates for Appropriations Committees*, p. 252).

[42] An example of these arguments can be found *in Threat to Title X and Other Women's Health Services*, pp. 22-35.

[43] *Family Planning Annual Report: 2007 National Summary*, p. 9.

[44] An example of these arguments can be found in *Threat to Title X and Other Women's Health Services*, pp. 22-35.

[45] Email correspondence between the author and Maurice Huguley, Office of the Assistant Secretary for Legislation, U.S. Department of Health and Human Services, January 27, 2009. See also the discussion of publicly funded family planning services in "Programs to Reduce Unintended Pregnancy," in The Institute of Medicine, *The Best Intentions: Unintended Pregnancy and the Well-Being of Children and Families* (Washington: National Academy Press, 1995), p. 220, http://www.nap.edu/catalog.php?record_id=4903.

[46] An example of these arguments can be found in *Threat to Title X and Other Women's Health Services*, pp. 16-21. See also Jacqueline E. Darroch, et al., "Differences in Teenage Pregnancy Rates Among Five Developed Countries: The Roles of Sexual Activity and Contraceptive Use," *Family Planning Perspectives*, vol. 33, no. 6 (November/December 2001), pp. 244-251.

[47] U.S. General Accounting Office, *Federal Funds: Fiscal Year 2001 Expenditures by Selected Organizations Involved in Health-Related Activities*, GAO-03-527R, May 16, 2003, http://www.gao.gov/cgi-bin/getrpt?GAO-03-527R. This report has not been updated.

[48] Planned Parenthood Federation of America, *Planned Parenthood Services*,http://www.plannedparenthood.org/issues-action/birth-control/access-to-condoms/reports/pp-services-17317.htm.

[49] U.S. Department of Health and Human Services, "Ensuring Department of Health and Human Services Funds Do Not Support Coercive or Discriminatory Policies or Practices in Violation of Federal Law," 73 *Federal Register* 78072–78101, December 19, 2008, http://edocket.access.gpo.gov/2008/pdf/E8-30134.pdf.

[50] 73 *Federal Register* 78096-78097, §88.1.

[51] 73 *Federal Register* 79097, 79098, §88.3(g)(1), §88.4(d)(1).

[52] 73 *Federal Register* 78097, §88.2.

[53] 73 *Federal Register*78097, 78098, §88.3(c), §88.4(b)(2).

[54] 73 *Federal Register*78097, 78098, §88.3(f)(1), §88.4(c)(1).

[55] 73 *Federal Register* 78098-78101.

[56] 73 *Federal Register* 78072.

[57] Comments may be viewed at http://www.regulations.gov/fdmspublic/component/main?main=DocketDetail&d=HHS-OS-2008-0011.

[58] 42 C.F.R. 59.5(a)(5). Examples of such comments include Letter from Sharon L. Camp, President and CEO, Guttmacher Institute, to DHHS, September 24, 2008, http://www.guttmacher.org/media/resources/2008/09/24/GuttmacherInstitute-re-ConscienceRegulation.pdf, and Letter from Caroline Fredrickson, Director, Washington Legislative Office, American Civil Liberties Union (ACLU), Louise Melling, Director,

Reproductive Freedom Project, ACLU, and Vania Leveille, Washington Legislative Office, ACLU, et al. to DHHS, September 25, 2008, http://www.aclu.org/images/asset_upload_ file467_36942.pdf.

[59] 73 *Federal Register* 78087.

[60] 73 *Federal Register* 78077.

[61] 73 *Federal Register* 78084-78085.

[62] 73 *Federal Register* 78071-78072.

In: Nonmarital Childbearing: Trends,...   ISBN: 978-1-60741-756-9
Editor: Gilberto de la Rayes   © 2010 Nova Science Publishers, Inc.

Chapter 4

BIRTHS: PRELIMINARY DATA FOR 2007[*]

Brady E. Hamilton, Joyce A. Martin
and Stephanie J. Ventura

ABSTRACT

Objectives

This chapter presents preliminary data for 2007 on births in the United States. U.S. data on births are shown by age, live-birth order, race, and Hispanic origin of mother. Data on marital status, cesarean delivery, preterm births, and low birthweight are also presented.

Methods

Data in this chapter are based on 98.7 percent of births for 2007. The records are weighted to independent control counts of all births received in state vital statistics offices in 2007. Comparisons are made with 2006 data.

---

[*] This is an edited, reformatted and augmented version of a U. S. Department of Health and Human Services publication dated March 2009.

Results

The preliminary estimate of births in 2007 rose 1 percent to 4,317,119, the highest number of births ever registered for the United States. The general fertility rate increased by 1 percent in 2007, to 69.5 births per 1,000 women aged 15–44 years, the highest level since 1990. Increases occurred within all race and Hispanic origin groups and for nearly all age groups. The birth rate for U.S. teenagers 15–19 years rose again in 2007 by about 1 percent, to 42.5 births per 1,000. The birth rate for teenagers 15–17 and 18–19 years each increased by 1 percent in 2007, to 22.2 and 73.9 per 1,000, respectively. The rate for the youngest group, 10–14 years, was unchanged. Birth rates also increased for women in their twenties, thirties, and early forties between 2006 and 2007. The 2007 total fertility rate increased to 2,122.5 births per 1,000 women. All measures of childbearing by unmarried women rose to historic levels in 2007, with the number of births, birth rate, and proportion of births to unmarried women increasing 3 to 5 percent. The cesarean delivery rate rose 2 percent in 2007, to 31.8 percent, marking the 11th consecutive year of increase and another record high for the United States. The rate of preterm births (infants delivered at less than 37 weeks of gestation) decreased 1 percent in 2007, to 12.7 percent, with the decline predominately among infants born late preterm (at 34–36 weeks). The rate of low birthweight (less than 2,500 grams) also declined slightly in 2007, to 8.2 percent.

Keywords: births • birth rates • maternal and infant health • vital statistics

INTRODUCTION

This report from the Centers for Disease Control and Prevention's National Center for Health Statistics (NCHS) presents preliminary data on births and birth rates and selected maternal and infant health characteristics for the United States in 2007 (Tables 1–15). The findings are based on 98.7 percent of registered vital records occurring in calendar year 2007, which were received and processed by NCHS as of July 17, 2008. Trends in the preliminary reports for 1995–2006 births were confirmed by the final vital statistics for each year (1,2).

State-specific detailed tables for 2007 births showing the percentages of births to women under age 20 years, to unmarried women, delivered by cesarean, delivered preterm, and of low birthweight (based on preliminary data) are also presented in this report (Tables 11–15).

RESULTS

Births and Birth Rates

Key findings, illustrated in Tables 1–7 and Figures 1 and 2, show:

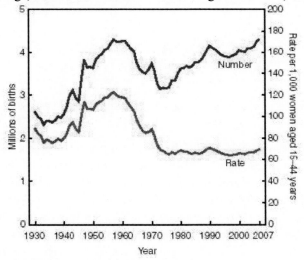

Source: CDC/NCHS, National Vital Statistics System.
Note: Beginning with 1959, trend lines are based on registered live births; trend lines for 1930–1958 are based on live births adjusted for underregistration.

Figure 1. Live births and fertility rates: United States, final 1930–2006 and preliminary 2007

- The preliminary **estimate of births** in 2007 was 4,317,119, 1 percent more than in 2006 (4,265,555) and the highest number ever registered for the United States (Tables 1 and 2; Figure 1) (1). This number surpasses the peak of the postwar "baby boom," in 1957 (3). Births rose for each race and Hispanic origin group, with increases ranging from less than 1 percent for non-Hispanic white women to 6 percent for Asian or Pacific Islander (API) women. Births to non-Hispanic black and Hispanic women each increased by nearly 2 percent.

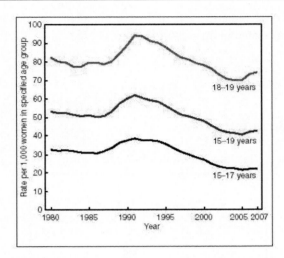

Figure 2. Birth rates for teenagers by age: United States, final 1980–2006 and preliminary 2007

- The preliminary **crude birth rate** (CBR) increased by nearly 1 percent in 2007 to 14.3 births per 1,000 total population from 14.2 in 2006. The **general fertility rate** (GFR) also increased in 2007, by 1 percent, to 69.5 births per 1,000 women aged 15–44 years, the highest level since 1990 (Figure 1) (1). The GFR rose for each race and Hispanic origin group, with increases ranging from less than 1 percent for Hispanic women to 6 percent for API women. The rates for non-Hispanic white and non-Hispanic black women, the two largest groups, each increased 1 percent.
- The **birth rate for U.S. teenagers** rose about 1 percent in 2007 (preliminary data). The rate in 2007 was 42.5 births per 1,000 teenagers 15–19 years, up from 41.9 in 2006 and 40.5 in 2005 (Tables 2–5; Figure 2). The teenage birth rate increased 5 percent between 2005 and 2007, with most of the increase occurring from 2005 to 2006. The recent increases have interrupted the 34 percent decline that extended from the peak in 1991 to 2005 (1).

  Among teenagers (under 20 years), only the rate for the youngest group, 10–14 years, was unchanged, at 0.6 births per 1,000. The number of births to this age group fell 3 percent, reflecting the declining number of females aged 10–14 years.

  The birth rate for teenagers 15–17 years increased about 1 percent to 22.2 per 1,000. This rate rose 4 percent from 2005 to 2007, interrupting the 45 percent decline reported for 1991–2005 (1). The number of infants born to this age group rose to 140,640 in 2007, up 1 percent from 2006 and 5 percent from 2005.

The birth rate for older teenagers rose 1 percent in 2007, to 73.9 per 1,000 aged 18–19 years. The 2007 rate was 6 percent higher than in 2005; these increases mark a halt, at least temporarily, in the long-term decline of 26 percent from 1991 to 2005.

Among race and Hispanic origin groups, the largest single-year increase was reported for American Indian or Alaska Native (AIAN) teenagers: The birth rate for this group rose 7 percent during 2006–2007, to 59.0 per 1,000 aged 15–19 years. This rate increased 12 percent from 2005 to 2007. The rates for non-Hispanic white and black teenagers and API teenagers each increased 1 to 2 percent. Only the rate for Hispanic teenagers declined in 2007, to 81.7 per 1,000, or 2 percent less than in 2006.

- The preliminary birth rate for women aged 20–24 years increased slightly (less than 1 percent) in 2007, to 106.4 births per 1,000 women from 105.9 (Tables 2 and 4–5). The *number of births* to women aged 20–24 years rose slightly between 2006 and 2007 (less than 1 percent), due entirely to the increased birth rate. The rate for women aged 25–29 years also increased in 2007, by 1 percent, to 117.5 births per 1,000 women from 116.7 in 2006. The number of births to women aged 25–29 years rose 2 percent in 2007, entirely a result of the increased birth rate.

- The preliminary birth rate for women aged 30–34 years increased in 2007 as well, by 2 percent, to 99.9 births per 1,000 women from 97.7 in 2006. This was the highest rate reported since 1964 (103.4), the end of the postwar "baby boom" (1946 to 1964) (1,3). The number of births to women aged 30–34 years increased 1 percent in 2007. The rate for women aged 35–39 years also increased in 2007, by less than 1 percent, to 47.5 births per 1,000 from 47.3 in 2006. This is the 29th consecutive year of increase as well as the highest rate over the past 40 years (49.9 in 1964) (1,3). The number of births to women aged 35–39 years increased slightly between 2006 and 2007.

- The preliminary birth rate for women aged 40–44 years increased 1 percent in 2007, to 9.5 births per 1,000 women, the highest rate since 1968 (9.6); the rate for women aged 45–49 years (which includes births to women aged 50–54 years) was unchanged at 0.6 births per 1,000 (Tables 2, 4, and 5). The number of births to women aged 40–

44 years decreased slightly, whereas the number of births to women aged 45–54 years increased 5 percent.

- The preliminary estimate of the **total fertility rate** (TFR) in 2007 was 2,122.5 births per 1,000 women, a 1 percent increase compared with the rate in 2006 (2,100.5, see Table 1). The TFR summarizes the potential impact of current fertility patterns on completed family size by estimating the average number of births that a hypothetical group of 1,000 women would have over their lifetimes, based on age-specific birth rates observed in the given year.

  The U.S. TFR in 2007 marks the second consecutive year in which the rate has been above replacement. A replacement rate is the rate at which a given generation can exactly replace itself, generally considered to be 2,100 births per 1,000 women. The TFR had been below replacement from 1972 through 2005. The TFR by race and Hispanic origin rose significantly in 2007 for all groups, with increases ranging from less than 1 percent for non-Hispanic white women to 6 percent for API women (Table 1).

- The preliminary first-birth rate for women aged 15–44 years increased 2 percent in 2007, to 27.9 births per 1,000 from 27.4 in 2006 (Table 5) (1). First-birth rates for women in age groups 15–34 years increased in 2007 by 1 to 2 percent; rates for women in the remaining age groups were unchanged. The rates for second-, third-, and fourth- and higher-order births for women aged 15–44 years increased in 2007 by 1 percent each.

- Preliminary **CBRs for states** varied considerably in 2007, ranging from 10.5 births per 1,000 total population in Vermont to 20.8 in Utah (Table 6). Birth rates for 13 states (Alabama, California, Indiana, Kansas, Kentucky, Louisiana, New Jersey, New York, Ohio, Pennsylvania, Texas, Washington, and West Virginia) increased significantly between 2006 and 2007, whereas birth rates for three states (Arizona, Colorado, and Michigan) and three territories (American Samoa, Puerto Rico, and Northern Marianas) decreased significantly. The rates for the remaining states, District of Columbia, and U.S. Virgin Islands were essentially unchanged (i.e., not statistically different).

  GFRs for states varied considerably in 2007 as well, ranging from 53.2 births per 1,000 women age 15–44 years in Vermont to 94.4 in Utah (Table 6). Fertility rates increased significantly for 30 states between 2006 and 2007 (Alabama, California, Florida, Georgia,

Hawaii, Idaho, Illinois, Indiana, Iowa, Kansas, Kentucky, Louisiana, Maryland, Minnesota, Mississippi, Missouri, Nevada, New Jersey, New Mexico, New York, North Carolina, Ohio, Oklahoma, Pennsylvania, Tennessee, Texas, Virginia, Washington, West Virginia, and Wisconsin). However, fertility rates for three territories only (American Samoa, Puerto Rico, and Northern Marianas) decreased significantly. Fertility rates for the remaining states, District of Columbia, and U.S. Virgin Islands were essentially unchanged.

- All measures of **childbearing by unmarried women** increased in the United States to historic levels in 2007 (preliminary data) (1,4). The total number of births to unmarried women increased 4 percent from 2006, to 1,714,643 (Table 7). The 2007 total is up 26 percent from 2002 when the recent steep increases began. Births to unmarried women increased from 2006 to 2007 within each age group 15 years and over, and the increases far outpaced those in total (married and unmarried) births for ages 15–39 years, the principal childbearing years. Nonmarital births to 10–14 year olds declined 2 percent.

- The preliminary birth rate for unmarried women rose 5 percent percent in 2007 to 52.9 births per 1,000 unmarried women aged 15–44 years. This rate has increased 21 percent since 2002 (43.7), following several years of relative stability.

- The preliminary proportion of all births to unmarried women increased to 39.7 percent in 2007, up from 38.5 percent in 2006. This proportion increased for all race and Hispanic origin population groups (Tables 1 and 7).

- The largest increases in numbers of nonmarital births were reported for women aged 25–39 years; these increases amounted to 6 percent or more for 2006–2007.

- Teenagers accounted for 23 percent of all nonmarital births in 2007, continuing a steady decline measured over the last several decades. In 1975, teenage mothers comprised 52 percent of nonmarital births (4).

- In 2007, about six in seven births to teenagers were non-marital. Sixty percent of births to women aged 20–24 years and almost one-third of births to women aged 25–29 years were to unmarried women (Table 7).

Maternal and Infant Health Birth Characteristics

Key findings, illustrated in Tables 8 and 9 and Figures 3 and 4, show:

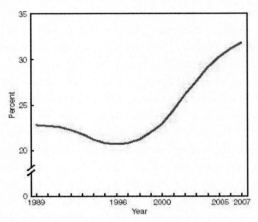

Source: CDC/NCHS, National Vital Statistics System.
Note: The total cesarean delivery rate is the percentage of all live births by cesarean
   delivery.

Figure 3. Total cesarean delivery rate: United States, final 1989–2006 and preliminary
2007

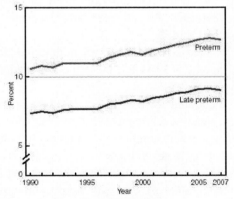

Source: CDC/NCHS, National Vital Statistics System.
Note: Preterm is less than 37 completed weeks of gestation. Late preterm is 34–36
   completed weeks of gestation.

Figure 4. Preterm birth rates: United States, final 1990–2006 and preliminary 2007

Table 1. Total Births and Percentage of Births with Selected Demographic Characteristics, by Race and Hispanic Origin of Mother: United States, Final 2006 and Preliminary 2007

[Data for 2007 are based on a continuous file of records received from the states. Figures for 2007 are based on weighted data rounded to the nearest individual. Birth rates are live births per 1,000 population in the specified group. Fertility rates are live births per 1,000 women aged 15–44 years in the specified group. Total fertility rates are sums of birth rates for 5-year age groups in the specified group, multiplied by 5]

Race and Hispanic origin of mother	Number of births		Birth rate		Fertility rate		Total fertility rate		Percent of births to unmarried women	
	2007	2006	2007	2006	2007	2006	2007	2006	2007	2006
All races and origins[1]	4,317,119	4,265,555	14.3	14.2	69.5	68.5	2,122.5	2,100.5	39.7	38.5
Non-Hispanic white[2]	2,312,473	2,308,640	11.5	11.6	60.1	59.5	1,871.0	1,863.5	27.8	26.6
Non-Hispanic black[2]	627,230	617,247	16.4	16.5	71.6	70.6	2,134.5	2,115.0	71.6	70.7
American Indian or Alaska Native total[2,3]	49,284	47,721	15.2	14.9	64.7	63.1	1,860.5	1,829.0	65.2	64.6
Asian or Pacific Islander total[2,3]	254,734	241,045	17.2	16.6	71.4	67.5	2,043.0	1,919.0	16.9	16.5
Hispanic[4]	1,061,970	1,039,077	23.3	23.4	102.1	101.5	2,992.0	2,959.5	51.3	49.9

[1] Includes origin not stated.

[2] Race and Hispanic origin are reported separately on birth certificates. Persons of Hispanic origin may be of any race. (OMB) standards. In 2007, 27 states reported multiple-race data. The multiple-race data for these states were bridged other states; see "Technical Notes." Multiple-race reporting areas vary for 2006–2007; see "Technical Notes."

[3] Data for persons of Hispanic origin are included for this race group; see "Technical Notes."

[4] Includes all persons of Hispanic origin of any race; see "Technical Notes."

Note: For information on the relative standard errors of the data and further discussion, see reference 5.

- The preliminary cesarean delivery rate rose 2 percent in 2007, to 31.8 percent of all births, marking the 11th consecutive year of increase and another record high for the United States (Table 8; Figure 3). This rate has climbed by more than 50 percent over the last decade (20.7 percent in 1996). Increases between 2006 and 2007 in the percentage of births delivered by cesarean were reported for most age groups (data not shown), and for the three largest race and Hispanic origin groups: non-Hispanic white (32.0 percent in 2007), non-Hispanic black (33.8 percent) and Hispanic (30.4 percent). The rise in the total cesarean delivery rate in recent years has been shown to result from higher rates of both first and repeat cesareans (1).

Table 2. Births and Birth Rates, by Age and Race and Hispanic Origin of Mother: United States, Final 2006 and Preliminary 2007

[Data for 2007 are based on a continuous file of records received from the states. Figures for 2007 are based on weighted data rounded to the nearest individual, so categories may not add to totals. Rates are per 1,000 women in the specified age and race and Hispanic origin group]

Age and race and Hispanic origin of mother	2007		2006	
	Number of births	Rate	Number of births	Rate
All races and origins[1]				
Total[2]	4,317,119	69.5	4,265,555	68.5
10–14 years	6,218	0.6	6,396	0.6
15–19 years	445,045	42.5	435,436	41.9
15–17 years	140,640	22.2	138,943	22.0
18–19 years	304,405	73.9	296,493	73.0
20–24 years	1,082,837	106.4	1,080,437	105.9
25–29 years	1,208,504	117.5	1,181,899	116.7
30–34 years	962,179	99.9	950,258	97.7
35–39 years	499,916	47.5	498,616	47.3
40–44 years	105,071	9.5	105,539	9.4
45–54 years[3]	7,349	0.6	6,974	0.6
Non-Hispanic white[4]				
Total[2]	2,312,473	60.1	2,308,640	59.5
10–14 years	1,269	0.2	1,267	0.2
15–19 years	173,104	27.2	169,729	26.6
15–17 years	45,144	11.8	45,260	11.8

Age and race and Hispanic origin of mother	2007		2006	
	Number of births	Rate	Number of births	Rate
18–19 years	127,960	50.5	124,469	49.3
20–24 years	526,943	83.3	528,355	83.4
25–29 years	676,599	108.8	665,479	109.1
30–34 years	566,197	99.7	566,708	98.1
35–39 years	301,666	45.8	309,033	46.3
40–44 years	62,152	8.6	63,590	8.4
45–54 years[3]	4,544	0.6	4,479	0.6
Non-Hispanic black[4]				
Total[2]	627,230	71.6	617,247	70.6
10–14 years	2,326	1.5	2,462	1.6
15–19 years	106,224	64.3	103,725	63.7
15–17 years	36,266	35.8	36,365	36.2
18–19 years	69,958	109.3	67,360	108.4
20–24 years	200,273	133.6	198,733	133.2
25–29 years	157,173	107.5	153,613	107.1
30–34 years	97,332	74.4	95,781	72.6
35–39 years	50,614	36.4	49,927	36.0
40–44 years	12,428	8.6	12,268	8.3
45–54 years[3]	860	0.6	738	0.5
American Indian or Alaska Native total[4,5]				
Total[2]	49,284	64.7	47,721	63.1
10–14 years	120	0.9	124	0.9
15–19 years	8,925	59.0	8,261	55.0
15–17 years	2,909	31.7	2,820	30.7
18–19 years	6,016	101.3	5,441	93.0
20–24 years	16,759	116.3	16,447	115.4
25–29 years	12,420	96.4	12,198	97.8
30–34 years	7,052	63.7	6,780	61.8
35–39 years	3,265	29.4	3,143	28.4
40–44 years	704	6.1	726	6.1
45–54 years[3]	38	0.3	42	0.4
Asian or Pacific Islander total[4,5]				
Total[2]	254,734	71.4	241,045	67.5
10–14 years	92	0.2	73	0.2
15–19 years	8,022	17.3	7,812	17.0

Table 2. (Continued)

Age and race and Hispanic origin of mother	2007 Number of births	Rate	2006 Number of births	Rate
15–17 years	2,336	8.4	2,438	8.8
18–19 years	5,686	30.7	5,374	29.5
20–24 years	32,309	66.2	31,860	63.2
25–29 years	71,465	117.9	66,913	108.4
30–34 years	86,949	125.1	82,885	116.9
35–39 years	46,379	66.3	42,394	63.0
40–44 years	8,879	14.5	8,549	14.1
45–54 years[3]	639	1.1	559	1.0
Hispanic[6]				
Total[2]	1,061,970	102.1	1,039,077	101.5
10–14 years	2,407	1.2	2,456	1.3
15–19 years	148,453	81.7	145,669	83.0
15–17 years	53,941	47.8	51,990	47.9
18–19 years	94,511	137.1	93,679	139.7
20–24 years	305,107	178.5	303,454	177.0
25–29 years	287,730	155.6	280,615	152.4
30–34 years	201,212	110.8	194,594	108.5
35–39 years	95,694	56.4	91,568	55.6
40–44 years	20,273	13.4	19,700	13.3
45–54 years[3]	1,095	0.8	1,021	0.8

[1] Includes origin not stated.

[2] The total number includes births to women of all ages, 10–54 years. The rate shown for all ages is the fertility rate, which is defined as the total number of births (regardless of the mother's age) per 1,000 women aged 15–44 years.

[3] The total number includes births to women aged 45–54 years. The birth rate for women aged 45–49 years is computed by relating the number of births to women aged 45–54 years to women aged 45–49 years, because most of the births in this group are to women aged 45–49 years.

[4] Race and Hispanic origin are reported separately on birth certificates. Persons of Hispanic origin may be of any race. Race categories are consistent with the 1977 Office of Management and Budget (OMB) standards. In 2007, 27 states reported multiple-race data. The multiple-race data for these states were bridged to the single-race categories of the 1977 OMB standards for comparability with other states; see "Technical Notes." Multiple-race reporting areas vary for 2006–2007; see "Technical Notes."

[5] Data for persons of Hispanic origin are included for this race group; see "Technical Notes."

[6] Includes all persons of Hispanic origin of any race; see "Technical Notes."

Note: For information on the relative standard errors of the data and further discussion, see reference 5.

Table 3. Birth Rates for Women Aged 15–19 Years, by Age and Race and Hispanic Origin of Mother: United States, Final 1991, 2005, and 2006, and Preliminary 2007; and Percentage of Change in Rates, 1991–2005, 2005–2007, and 2006–2007

[Data for 2007 are based on a continuous file of records received from the states. Rates are per 1,000 women in the specified age and race and Hispanic origin group]

Age and race and Hispanic origin of mother	Year				Percent change		
	2007	2006	2005	1991	2006–2007	2005–2007	1991–2005
10–14 years							
All races and origins[1]	0.6	0.6	0.7	1.4	0	−14	−50
Non-Hispanic white[2]	0.2	0.2	0.2	0.5	0	0	−60
Non-Hispanic black[2]	1.5	1.6	1.7	4.9	−6	−12	−65
American Indian or Alaska Native total[2,3] .	0.9	0.9	0.9	1.6	0	0	−44
Asian or Pacific Islander total[2,3]	0.2	0.2	0.2	0.8	0	0	−75
Hispanic[4]	1.2	1.3	1.3	2.4	−8	−8	−46
15–19 years							
All races and origins[1]	42.5	41.9	40.5	61.8	1	5	−34
Non-Hispanic white[2]	27.2	26.6	25.9	43.4	2	5	−40
Non-Hispanic black[2]	64.3	63.7	60.9	118.2	1	6	−48
American Indian or Alaska Native total[2,3] .	59.0	55.0	52.7	84.1	7	12	−37
Asian or Pacific Islander total[2,3]	17.3	17.0	17.0	27.3	2	2	−38
Hispanic[4]	81.7	83.0	81.7	104.6	−2	0	−22
15–17 years							
All races and origins[1]	22.2	22.0	21.4	38.6	1	4	−45
Non-Hispanic white[2]	11.8	11.8	11.5	23.6	0	3	−51
Non-Hispanic black[2]	35.8	36.2	34.9	86.1	−1	3	−59
American Indian or Alaska Native total[2,3]	31.7	30.7	30.5	51.9	3	4	−41
Asian or Pacific Islander total[2,3]	8.4	8.8	8.2	16.3	−5	2	−50

Table 3. (Continued)

Age and race and Hispanic origin of mother	Year				Percent change		
	2007	2006	2005	1991	2006–2007	2005–2007	1991–2005
Hispanic[4]	47.8	47.9	48.5	69.2	0	−1	−30
18–19 years							
All races and origins[1]	73.9	73.0	69.9	94.0	1	6	−26
Non-Hispanic white[2]	50.5	49.3	48.0	70.6	2	5	−32
Non-Hispanic black[2]	109.3	108.4	103.0	162.2	1	6	−36
American Indian or Alaska Native total[2,3] . .	101.3	93.0	87.6	134.2	9	16	−35
Asian or Pacific Islander total[2,3]	30.7	29.5	30.1	42.2	4	2	−29
Hispanic[4]	137.1	139.7	134.6	155.5	−2	2	−13

[1] Includes origin not stated.

[2] Race and Hispanic origin are reported separately on birth certificates. Persons of Hispanic origin may be of any race. (OMB) standards. In 2007, 27 states reported multiple-race data. The multiple-race data for these states were bridged other states; see "Technical Notes." Multiple-race reporting areas vary for 2005–2007; see "Technical Notes."

[3] Data for persons of Hispanic origin are included for this race group; see "Technical Notes."

[4] Includes all persons of Hispanic origin of any race; see "Technical Notes."

Note: For information on the relative standard errors of the data and further discussion, see reference 5.

Table 4. Live Births by Age of Mother, Live-Birth Order, and Race and Hispanic Origin of Mother: United States, Preliminary 2007

[Data are based on a continuous file of records received from the states. Figures are based on weighted data rounded to the nearest individual, so categories may not add to totals]

Live-birth order and race and Hispanic origin of mother	All ages	Age of mother							
		Under 15 years	15-19 years	20-24 years	25-29 years	30-34 years	35-39 years	40-44 years	45-54 years
All races and origins[1]	4,317,119	6,218	445,045	1,082,837	1,208,504	962,179	499,916	105,071	7,349
1st child	1,726,523	6,088	357,092	524,240	432,011	270,057	112,833	22,322	1,881
2d child	1,364,048	99	73,891	359,732	400,000	334,881	163,927	29,721	1,797
3d child	722,883	2	10,863	141,942	230,640	201,033	114,878	22,220	1,307
4th child and over	483,766	1	1,472	52,063	140,490	151,655	105,601	30,175	2,310
Not stated	19,897	29	1,727	4,861	5,364	4,552	2,677	634	54
Non-Hispanic white[2]	2,312,473	1,269	173,104	526,943	676,599	566,197	301,666	62,152	4,544
1st child	967,305	1,251	144,966	278,691	276,142	175,213	74,888	14,837	1,317
2d child	760,952	14	24,353	170,681	228,865	210,811	105,975	19,065	1,190
3d child	364,534	–	2,889	58,493	112,351	109,632	67,613	12,775	780
4th child and over .	210,171	–	316	17,048	56,656	68,090	51,682	15,149	1,228
Not stated	9,511	5	581	2,029	2,585	2,451	1,508	325	28

Table 4. (Continued)

| | | Age of mother | | | | | | | |
Live-birth order and race and Hispanic origin of mother	All ages	Under 15 years	15–19 years	20–24 years	25–29 years	30–34 years	35–39 years	40–44 years	45–54 years
Non-Hispanic black[2]	627,230	2,326	106,224	200,273	157,173	97,332	50,614	12,428	860
1st child	243,684	2,264	83,138	86,025	40,096	20,335	9,437	2,214	175
2d child	177,902	48	18,645	65,267	48,480	28,218	13,919	3,140	185
3d child	107,439	–	3,281	31,938	35,608	22,166	11,656	2,642	147
4th child and over .	93,841	1	538	15,700	31,867	25,851	15,224	4,315	344
Not stated	4,365	13	622	1,343	1,123	762	377	117	8
American Indian or Alaska Native total[2,3]	49,284	120	8,925	16,759	12,420	7,052	3,265	704	38
1st child	17,606	119	6,844	6,538	2,559	1,058	407	79	3
2d child	13,270	1	1,743	5,690	3,468	1,632	627	103	6
3d child	8,792		266	3,075	3,068	1,586	673	123	1
4th child and over	9,406	–	37	1,392	3,269	2,743	1,546	390	28
Not stated	211	–	34	65	56	34	12	9	–
Asian or Pacific Islander total[2,3]	254,734	92	8,022	32,309	71,465	86,949	46,379	8,879	639
1st child	116,225	90	6,509	19,338	38,963	35,491	13,343	2,293	198
2d child	89,426	1	1,232	8,797	21,681	35,129	19,265	3,134	188
3d child	31,617		199	2,875	6,902	10,770	8,870	1,894	107

Table 4. (Continued)

Live-birth order and race and Hispanic origin of mother	All ages	Age of mother							
		Under 15 years	15–19 years	20–24 years	25–29 years	30–34 years	35–39 years	40–44 years	45–54 years
4th child and over	16,372	–	30	1,116	3,632	5,237	4,704	1,514	139
Not stated	1,093	1	53	183	286	322	197	44	7
Hispanic[4]	1,061,970	2,407	148,453	305,107	287,730	201,212	95,694	20,273	1,095
1st child	377,282	2,361	115,346	132,872	72,881	36,730	14,162	2,760	171
2d child	319,355	35	27,923	109,057	96,688	57,956	23,390	4,111	196
3d child	209,148	2	4,247	45,437	72,342	56,467	25,745	4,676	231
4th child and over	152,705	–	550	16,745	44,842	49,374	32,048	8,653	493
Not stated	3,481	9	387	997	976	685	350	74	3

– Quantity zero.

[1] Includes origin not stated.

[2] Race and Hispanic origin are reported separately on birth certificates. Persons of Hispanic origin may be of any race. (OMB) standards. In 2007, 27 states reported multiple-race data. The multiple-race data for these states were bridged other states; see "Technical Notes."

[3] Data for persons of Hispanic origin are included for this race group; see "Technical Notes."

[4] Includes all persons of Hispanic origin of any race; see "Technical Notes."

Note: For information on the relative standard errors of the data and further discussion, see reference 5.

Table 5. Birth Rates by Age of Mother, Live-Birth Order, and Race and Hispanic Origin of Mother: United States, Preliminary 2007

[Data are based on a continuous file of records received from the states. Rates are per 1,000 women in the specified age and race and Hispanic origin group]

Live-birth order and race and Hispanic origin of mother	Age of mother								
	15-44 years[1]	10-14 years	15-19 years	20-24 years	25-29 years	30-34 years	35-39 years	40-44 years	45-49 years[2]
All races and origins[3]	69.5	0.6	42.5	106.4	117.5	99.9	47.5	9.5	0.6
1st child	27.9	0.6	34.2	51.7	42.2	28.2	10.8	2.0	0.2
2d child	22.1	0.0	7.1	35.5	39.1	35.0	15.7	2.7	0.2
3d child	11.7	*	1.0	14.0	22.5	21.0	11.0	2.0	0.1
4th child and over	7.8	*	0.1	5.1	13.7	15.8	10.1	2.8	0.2
Non-Hispanic white[4]	60.1	0.2	27.2	83.3	108.8	99.7	45.8	8.6	0.6
1st child	25.2	0.2	22.9	44.2	44.5	31.0	11.4	2.1	0.2
2d child	19.9	*	3.9	27.1	36.9	37.2	16.2	2.6	0.2
3d child	9.5	*	0.5	9.3	18.2	19.4	10.3	1.8	0.1
4th child and over .	5.5	*	0.1	2.7	9.2	12.1	7.9	2.1	0.2
Non-Hispanic black[4]	71.6	1.5	64.3	133.6	107.5	74.4	36.4	8.6	0.6
1st child	28.0	1.5	50.6	57.8	27.6	15.7	6.8	1.5	0.1
2d child	20.4	0.0	11.4	43.8	33.4	21.7	10.1	2.2	0.1

Table 5. (Continued)

Live-birth order and race and Hispanic origin of mother	Age of mother								
	15–44 years[1]	10–14 years	15–19 years	20–24 years	25–29 years	30–34 years	35–39 years	40–44 years	45–49 years[2]
3d child	12.3	*	2.0	21.5	24.5	17.0	8.4	1.8	0.1
4th child and over .	10.8	*	0.3	10.5	22.0	19.9	11.0	3.0	0.2
American Indian or Alaska Native total[4,5]	64.7	0.9	59.0	116.3	96.4	63.7	29.4	6.1	0.3
1st child	23.2	0.9	45.5	45.6	19.9	9.6	3.7	0.7	*
2d child	17.5	*	11.6	39.7	27.0	14.8	5.7	0.9	*
3d child	11.6	*	1.8	21.4	23.9	14.4	6.1	1.1	*
4th child and over	12.4	*	0.2	9.7	25.5	24.9	14.0	3.4	0.2
Asian or Pacific Islander total[4,5]	71.4	0.2	17.3	66.2	117.9	125.1	66.3	14.5	1.1
1st child	32.7	0.2	14.1	39.8	64.5	51.3	19.2	3.7	0.4
2d child	25.2	*	2.7	18.1	35.9	50.7	27.7	5.1	0.3
3d child	8.9	*	0.4	5.9	11.4	15.6	12.7	3.1	0.2
4th child and over	4.6	*	0.1	2.3	6.0	7.6	6.8	2.5	0.2
Hispanic[6]	102.1	1.2	81.7	178.5	155.6	110.8	56.4	13.4	0.8
1st child	36.4	1.2	63.6	78.0	39.5	20.3	8.4	1.8	0.1
2d child	30.8	0.0	15.4	64.0	52.5	32.0	13.8	2.7	0.2
3d child	20.2	*	2.3	26.7	39.2	31.2	15.2	3.1	0.2
4th child and over	14.7	*	0.3	9.8	24.3	27.3	19.0	5.7	0.4

0.0 Quantity more than zero but less than 0.05.

* Figure does not meet standards of reliability or precision; based on fewer than 20 births in the numerator[1] The rate shown is the fertility rate, which is defined as the total number of births, regardless of age of mother, per 1,000 women aged 15–44 years.

[2] The birth rate for women aged 45–49 years is computed by relating births to women aged 45–54 years to women aged 45–49 years, because most of the births in this group are to women aged 45–49 years.

[3] Includes origin not stated.

[4] Race and Hispanic origin are reported separately on birth certificates. Persons of Hispanic origin may be of any race. Race categories are consistent with the 1977 Office of Management and Budget (OMB) standards. In 2007, 27 states reported multiple-race data. The multiple-race data for these states were bridged to the single-race categories of the 1977 OMB standards for comparability with other states; see "Technical Notes."

[5] Data for persons of Hispanic origin are included for this race group; see "Technical Notes."

[6] Includes all persons of Hispanic origin of any race; see "Technical Notes."

Note: For information on the relative standard errors of the data and further discussion, see reference 5.

Table 6. Live Births by Race and Hispanic Origin of Mother, and Birth and Fertility Rates: United States and Each State and Territory, Preliminary 2007

[By place of residence. Data are based on a continuous file of records received from the states. Figures are based on weighted data rounded to the nearest individual, so categories may not add to totals. Birth rates are total births per 1,000 total population; fertility rates are total births per 1,000 women aged 15–44 years]

Area	All races and origins[1]	Non-Hispanic white[2]	Number of births				Birth rate All races	Fertility rate All races
			Non-Hispanic black[2]	American Indian or Alaska Native total[2,3]	Asian or Pacific Islander total[2,3]	Hispanic[4]		
United States[5]	4,317,119	2,312,473	627,230	49,284	254,734	1,061,970	14.3	69.5
Alabama	64,749	38,464	19,740	189	942	5,391	14.0	68.7
Alaska	11,101	6,291	409	2,836	835	825	16.2	77.5

Table 6. (Continued)

Area	All races and origins[1]	Non-Hispanic white[2]	Non-Hispanic black[2]	American Indian or Alaska Native total[2,3]	Asian or Pacific Islander total[2,3]	Hispanic[4]	Birth rate All races	Fertility rate All races
				Number of births				
Arizona	102,992	42,521	3,914	6,700	3,597	46,373	16.2	81.1
Arkansas	41,377	27,720	8,080	261	721	4,515	14.6	73.1
California	566,352	155,930	31,777	3,626	74,292	296,942	15.5	72.5
Colorado	70,805	41,853	3,122	755	2,493	22,221	14.6	69.8
Connecticut	41,663	24,897	5,183	238	2,441	8,832	11.9	59.5
Delaware	12,171	6,494	3,215	16	530	1,912	14.1	68.4
District of Columbia	8,862	2,227	4,936	2	259	1,450	15.1	60.0
Florida	239,143	107,843	51,835	805	7,988	70,833	13.1	68.4
Georgia	152,021	70,735	49,278	437	5,696	24,319	15.9	73.7
Hawaii	19,137	4,557	426	77	12,958	3,007	14.9	76.0
Idaho	25,019	20,190	139	451	416	3,870	16.7	83.4
Illinois	180,856	95,508	31,655	262	9,212	44,151	14.1	67.4
Indiana	89,847	68,907	10,229	118	1,693	8,805	14.2	69.7
Iowa	40,885	34,521	1,804	315	1,021	3,355	13.7	70.1
Kansas	42,004	30,512	3,059	376	1,367	6,689	15.1	75.6
Kentucky	59,370	49,842	5,418	114	1,018	3,092	14.0	68.6
Louisiana	66,260	36,172	25,343	476	1,160	3,188	15.4	73.3
Maine	14,120	13,186	325	125	223	209	10.7	55.6
Maryland	78,096	36,128	26,198	151	5,484	10,608	13.9	65.6
Massachusetts	77,962	53,274	7,262	185	6,013	10,900	12.1	57.4
Michigan	125,394	85,528	22,343	765	4,337	8,441	12.4	61.5

Table 6. (Continued)

| Area | Number of births | | | | | | Birth rate All races | Fertility rate All races |
	All races and origins[1]	Non-Hispanic white[2]	Non-Hispanic black[2]	American Indian or Alaska Native total[2,3]	Asian or Pacific Islander total[2,3]	Hispanic[4]		
Minnesota	73,745	53,856	6,615	1,673	5,412	5,939	14.2	69.7
Mississippi	46,501	23,068	20,894	309	475	1,708	15.9	76.9
Missouri	81,928	62,211	12,610	435	1,978	4,667	13.9	68.8
Montana	12,444	9,623	62	1,599	145	372	13.0	68.6
Nebraska	26,923	20,008	1,794	618	754	4,068	15.2	76.2
Nevada	41,202	16,959	3,615	576	3,544	16,144	16.1	79.6
New Hampshire	14,169	12,620	203	54	540	593	10.8	53.8
New Jersey	116,060	56,139	17,863	188	11,944	30,027	13.4	66.1
New Mexico	30,555	8,662	522	3,835	1,330	17,007	15.5	76.4
New York	253,458	125,632	42,738	629	24,084	60,134	13.1	62.1
North Carolina	131,016	72,416	30,635	1,772	3,988	22,113	14.5	69.6
North Dakota	8,840	7,277	129	1,012	110	278	13.8	69.8
Ohio	150,882	115,583	24,222	320	3,291	6,611	13.2	65.5
Oklahoma	55,078	35,334	4,914	6,517	1,259	7,173	15.2	76.0
Oregon	49,372	34,256	1,145	955	2,712	10,133	13.2	66.1
Pennsylvania	150,731	107,818	21,281	407	6,260	13,793	12.1	61.9
Rhode Island	12,375	5,999	1,045	159	536	2,588	11.7	55.8
South Carolina	62,891	34,411	20,489	274	1,159	6,215	14.3	69.9
South Dakota	12,259	9,351	212	2,158	149	471	15.4	80.0
Tennessee	86,707	58,588	17,768	387	2,003	8,383	14.1	68.8
Texas	407,640	140,272	46,397	1,064	16,032	204,498	17.1	80.1
Utah	55,131	42,844	539	768	1,761	9,042	20.8	94.4

Table 6. (Continued)

Area	Number of births						Birth rate All races	Fertility rate All races
	All races and origins[1]	Non-Hispanic white[2]	Non-Hispanic black[2]	American Indian or Alaska Native total[2,3]	Asian or Pacific Islander total[2,3]	Hispanic[4]		
Vermont	6,513	6,178	95	14	91	78	10.5	53.2
Virginia	108,874	62,155	23,842	176	8,021	14,966	14.1	67.0
Washington	88,958	56,299	3,812	2,492	9,303	16,881	13.8	66.9
West Virginia	21,992	20,700	778	23	181	253	12.1	63.1
Wisconsin	72,796	54,549	7,240	1,255	2,895	6,934	13.0	65.0
Wyoming	7,893	6,361	79	333	79	969	15.1	77.7
Puerto Rico	46,636	1,381	115	- - -	- - -	45,123	11.8	55.2
Virgin Islands	1,674	125	1,139	82	–	270	15.2	74.0
Guam	- - -	- - -	- - -	- - -	- - -	- - -	- - -	- - -
American Samoa	1,288	- - -	- - -	–	1,288	- - -	20.1	90.5
Northern Marianas	1,345	- - -	- - -	–	1,327	- - -	15.9	38.8

- - - Data not available.

– Quantity zero.

[1] Includes origin not stated.

[2] Race and Hispanic origin are reported separately on birth certificates. Persons of Hispanic origin may be of any race. Race categories are consistent with the 1977 Office of Management and Budget (OMB) standards. In 2007, 27 states reported multiple-race data. The multiple-race data for these states were bridged to the single-race categories of the 1977 OMB standards for comparability with other states; see "Technical Notes."

[3] Data for persons of Hispanic origin are included for this race group; see "Technical Notes."

[4] Includes all persons of Hispanic origin of any race; see "Technical Notes."

[5] Excludes data for the territories.

Note: For information on the relative standard errors of the data and further discussion, see reference 5.

Table 7. Number and Percentage of Births to Unmarried Women, by Age: United States, Final 2006 and Preliminary 2007

[Data for 2007 are based on a continuous file of records received from the states. Figures for 2007 are based on weighted data rounded to the nearest individual, so categories may not add to total]

Age of mother	Number of births		Percent	
	2007	2006	2007	2006
All ages, unmarried	1,714,643	1,641,946	39.7	38.5
Under 20 years	386,702	372,876	85.7	84.4
Under 15 years	6,142	6,288	98.8	98.3
15–19 years	380,560	366,588	85.5	84.2
15–17 years	130,519	127,749	92.8	91.9
18–19 years	250,041	238,839	82.1	80.6
20–24 years	644,591	625,780	59.5	57.9
25–29 years	389,169	366,085	32.2	31.0
30–34 years	185,425	173,586	19.3	18.3
35–39 years	86,343	81,828	17.3	16.4
40–54 years	22,411	21,791	19.9	19.4

Note: For information on the relative standard errors of the data and further discussion, see reference 5.

- The preliminary **preterm birth rate** was 12.7 percent for 2007, a decline of 1 percent from the 2006 level of 12.8 percent (Table 8). The preterm rate (infants delivered at less than 37 weeks of gestation per 100 births) had generally been on the rise for more than two decades (1). The 2007 decline was predominately among those born at 34–36 weeks, or late preterm. The late preterm rate, which had climbed more than 25 percent since 1990, was down slightly between 2006 and 2007, from 9.1 to 9.0 percent (Table 9; Figure 4). The total preterm rate declined modestly among births to non-Hispanic white (11.7 to 11.5 percent) and non-Hispanic black (18.5 to 18.3 percent) mothers for 2006–2007, but was essentially unchanged among births to Hispanic women (12.3 percent for 2007).

Table 8. Total Births, Total Cesarean Delivery rate, Percentage of Live Births Preterm and Very Preterm, and Percentage of Live Births at Low and Very Low Birthweight, by Race and Hispanic Origin of Mother: United States, Final 2006 and Preliminary 2007

[Data for 2007 are based on a continuous file of records received from the states. Figures for 2007 are based on weighted data rounded to the nearest individual]

Race and Hispanic origin of mother	Number of births		Cesarean rate[1]		Preterm				Low birthweight			
					Total[2]		Very preterm[3]		Total[4]		Very low birthweight[5]	
	2007	2006	2007	2006	2007	2006	2007	2006	2007	2006	2007	2006
All races and origins[6]	4,317,119	4,265,555	31.8	31.1	12.7	12.8	2.0	2.0	8.2	8.3	1.5	1.5
Non-Hispanic white[7]	2,312,473	2,308,640	32.0	31.3	11.5	11.7	1.6	1.7	7.2	7.3	1.2	1.2
Non-Hispanic black[7]	627,230	617,247	33.8	33.1	18.3	18.5	4.1	4.1	13.8	14.0	3.2	3.2
American Indian or Alaska Native total[7,8]	49,284	47,721	27.7	27.5	13.9	14.2	2.1	2.1	7.5	7.5	1.3	1.3
Asian or Pacific Islander total[7,8]	254,734	241,045	31.4	30.6	10.9	10.9	1.5	1.5	8.1	8.1	1.1	1.1
Hispanic[9]	1,061,970	1,039,077	30.4	29.7	12.3	12.2	1.8	1.8	6.9	7.0	1.2	1.2

[1] All births by cesarean delivery per 100 live births.
[2] Less than 37 completed weeks of gestation.
[3] Less than 32 completed weeks of gestation.
[4] Less than 2,500 grams (5lb 8oz).
[5] Less than 1,500 grams (3lb 4oz).
[6] Includes origin not stated.
[7] Race and Hispanic origin are reported separately on birth certificates. Persons of Hispanic origin may be of any race. Race categories are consistent with the 1977 Office of Management and Budget (OMB) standards. In 2007, 27 states reported multiple-race data. The multiple-race data for these states were bridged to the single-race categories of the 1977 OMB standards for comparability with other states; see "Technical Notes." Multiple-race reporting areas vary for 2006–2007; see "Technical Notes."
[8] Data for persons of Hispanic origin are included for this race group; see "Technical Notes."
[9] Includes all persons of Hispanic origin of any race; see "Technical Notes."
Note: For information on the relative standard errors of the data and further discussion, see reference 5.

Table 9. Percentage of Preterm Births: United States, Final 1990, 2000, 2005, and 2006, and Preliminary 2007

[Data for 2007 are based on a continuous file of records received from the states]

Year	Total preterm[1]	Late preterm[2]	32–33 weeks	Less than 32 weeks
2007	12.66	9.03	1.59	2.04
2006	12.80	9.14	1.62	2.04
2005	12.73	9.09	1.60	2.03
2000	11.64	8.22	1.49	1.93
1990	10.61	7.30	1.40	1.92

[1] Preterm is less than 37 completed weeks of gestation.

[2] Late preterm is 34–36 completed weeks of gestation.

Note: For information on the relative standard errors of the data and further discussion, see reference 5.

Table 10. Total Count of Records and Percent Completeness of Preliminary File of Live Births: United States, Each State and Territory, Preliminary 2007

[By place of occurrence]

Area	Live births	
	Counts of records	Percent completeness
United States[1]	4,325,427	98.7
Alabama	63,997	100.0
Alaska	11,004	99.7
Arizona	103,811	100.0
Arkansas	40,168	100.0
California	567,527	100.0
Colorado	71,220	100.0
Connecticut	42,270	100.0
Delaware	12,527	99.9
District of Columbia	14,822	100.0
Florida	239,396	100.0
Georgia	153,190	86.4
Hawaii	19,151	100.0
Idaho	24,436	100.0
Illinois	177,470	100.0
Indiana	90,561	100.0

Table 10. (Continued)

Area	Live births	
	Counts of records	**Counts of records**
Iowa	40,988	100.0
Kansas	42,938	100.0
Kentucky	57,425	100.0
Louisiana	66,328	91.4
Maine	13,974	100.0
Maryland	74,941	100.0
Massachusetts	78,723	100.0
Michigan	124,270	80.2
Minnesota	73,610	100.0
Mississippi	45,510	100.0
Missouri	82,824	100.0
Montana	12,403	100.0
Nebraska	27,112	100.0
Nevada	40,784	99.7
New Hampshire	13,937	100.0
New Jersey	112,881	100.0
New Mexico	29,901	100.0
New York	255,441	100.0
New York excluding New York City	126,469	100.0
New York City	128,972	100.0
North Carolina	132,188	100.0
North Dakota	10,152	100.0
Ohio	151,353	100.0
Oklahoma	54,168	100.0
Oregon	49,870	100.0
Pennsylvania	150,021	100.0
Rhode Island	13,191	100.0
South Carolina	60,196	100.0
South Dakota	12,815	100.0
Tennessee	92,050	100.0
Texas	414,177	99.4
Utah	56,320	100.0
Vermont	6,210	100.0
Virginia	107,263	100.0

Table 10. (Continued)

Area	Live births	
	Counts of records	Counts of records
Washington	88,937	100.0
West Virginia	21,915	100.0
Wisconsin	71,744	100.0
Wyoming	7,317	100.0
Puerto Rico	46,748	100.0
Virgin Islands	1,779	82.5
Guam	3,501	71.9
American Samoa	1,288	99.9
Northern Marianas	1,379	100.0

[1] Excludesdatafortheterritories.

Note: Percent completeness = Number of records in preliminary file * 100

Count of records

Table 11. Percentage of Live Births to Mothers Under 20 Years of Age: United States, Each State and Territory, Final 2006 and Preliminary 2007

[By place of residence. Data are based on a continuous file of records received from the states]

Area	2007	2006
United States[1]	10.5	10.4
Alabama	13.6	13.8
Alaska	10.1	10.1
Arizona	12.7	12.7
Arkansas	14.6	14.8
California	9.5	9.5
Colorado	9.7	9.7
Connecticut	6.9	7.0
Delaware	10.4	10.7
District of Columbia	12.1	12.0
Florida	10.9	10.9
Georgia	12.2	12.1
Hawaii	8.5	8.6
Idaho	9.1	8.9
Illinois	10.1	10.0
Indiana	11.2	10.9

Table 11. (Continued)

Area	2007	2006
Iowa	8.7	8.7
Kansas	10.3	10.2
Kentucky	12.9	12.9
Louisiana	13.7	13.9
Maine	8.4	8.1
Maryland	8.9	8.8
Massachusetts	6.4	6.2
Michigan	10.1	9.8
Minnesota	7.1	7.0
Mississippi	17.1	16.5
Missouri	11.4	11.4
Montana	9.7	10.3
Nebraska	8.6	8.0
Nevada	10.8	10.9
New Hampshire	6.6	6.1
New Jersey	6.4	6.3
New Mexico	15.7	15.7
New York	7.0	7.1
North Carolina	11.7	11.7
North Dakota	8.0	7.4
Ohio	11.0	10.7
Oklahoma	13.9	13.6
Oregon	8.9	8.9
Pennsylvania	9.3	9.3
Rhode Island	9.7	9.2
South Carolina	13.4	13.4
South Dakota	9.8	9.5
Tennessee	13.2	13.0
Texas	13.5	13.5
Utah	6.9	6.6
Vermont	7.6	7.2
Virginia	8.6	8.6
Washington	8.4	8.3
West Virginia	12.5	12.5
Wisconsin	8.7	8.4

Table 11. (Continued)

Area	2007	2006
Wyoming	11.8	11.2
Puerto Rico	18.3	18.4
Virgin Islands	12.8	12.7
Guam	- - -	12.9
American Samoa	7.4	7.7
Northern Marianas	8.5	7.5

- - -Data not available.

[1] Excludes data for the territories.

Note: For information on the relative standard errors of the data and further discussion, see reference 5.

Table 12. Percentage of Live Births to Unmarried Mothers: United States, Each State and Territory, Final 2006 and Preliminary 2007

[By place of residence. Data are based on a continuous file of records received from the states]

Area	2007	2006
United States[1]	39.7	38.5
Alabama	38.4	36.6
Alaska	37.2	36.8
Arizona	45.2	44.0
Arkansas	43.4	41.8
California	38.9	37.6
Colorado	25.4	27.6
Connecticut	35.1	34.0
Delaware	46.9	45.5
District of Columbia	58.5	57.6
Florida	46.1	44.4
Georgia	43.3	42.4
Hawaii	36.9	36.0
Idaho	25.5	24.3
Illinois	40.1	38.7
Indiana	42.4	41.4
Iowa	34.3	33.8
Kansas	36.5	35.2
Kentucky	39.3	35.3
Louisiana	50.9	49.8
Maine	39.1	37.1

Table 12. (Continued)

Area	2007	2006
Maryland	40.9	39.7
Massachusetts	33.4	32.2
Michigan	39.4	38.3
Minnesota	32.7	31.7
Mississippi	53.7	52.8
Missouri	40.5	39.3
Montana	35.9	36.0
Nebraska	33.4	32.3
Nevada	42.0	41.3
New Hampshire	31.4	29.4
New Jersey	34.4	33.0
New Mexico	51.8	51.2
New York	40.7	40.0
North Carolina	41.2	40.1
North Dakota	32.6	31.7
Ohio	42.2	40.5
Oklahoma	41.3	40.9
Oregon	35.1	34.3
Pennsylvania	39.7	38.3
Rhode Island	44.0	40.5
South Carolina	46.6	45.6
South Dakota	38.4	37.1
Tennessee	42.8	41.4
Texas	40.7	39.4
Utah	19.6	18.8
Vermont	36.6	34.5
Virginia	35.2	33.8
Washington	33.2	31.9
West Virginia	40.3	37.9
Wisconsin	35.4	34.1
Wyoming	34.7	33.0
Puerto Rico	59.3	57.8
Virgin Islands	71.5	70.8
Guam	- - -	57.7
American Samoa	33.0	34.7
Northern Marianas	46.1	58.8

- - - Data not available.

[1] Excludes data for the territories.

Note: For information on the relative standard errors of the data and further discussion, see reference 5.

Table 13. Percentage Low Birthweight: United States, Each State and Territory, Final 2006 and Preliminary

[By place of residence. Data are based on a continuous file of records received from the states. Low birthweight is less than 2,500 grams]

Area	2007	2006
United States[1]	8.2	8.3
Alabama	10.4	10.5
Alaska	5.7	6.0
Arizona	7.1	7.1
Arkansas	9.1	9.2
California	6.9	6.8
Colorado	9.0	8.9
Connecticut	8.1	8.1
Delaware	9.3	9.3
District of Columbia	11.1	11.5
Florida	8.7	8.7
Georgia	9.1	9.6
Hawaii	8.0	8.1
Idaho	6.5	6.9
Illinois	8.5	8.6
Indiana	8.5	8.2
Iowa	6.8	6.9
Kansas	6.0	7.2
Kentucky	9.3	9.1
Louisiana	11.0	11.4
Maine	6.3	6.8
Maryland	9.1	9.4
Massachusetts	7.9	7.9
Michigan	8.2	8.4
Minnesota	6.7	6.5
Mississippi	12.3	12.4
Missouri	7.8	8.1
Montana	7.2	7.3
Nebraska	7.0	7.1
Nevada	8.2	8.3
New Hampshire	6.3	6.9
New Jersey	8.5	8.6
New Mexico	8.8	8.9
New York	8.2	8.3
North Carolina	9.2	9.1

Table 13. (Continued)

Area	2007	2006
North Dakota	6.3	6.7
Ohio	8.7	8.8
Oklahoma	8.2	8.3
Oregon	6.1	6.1
Pennsylvania	8.4	8.5
Rhode Island	8.0	8.0
South Carolina	10.1	10.1
South Dakota	7.0	7.0
Tennessee	9.4	9.6
Texas	8.4	8.4
Utah	6.7	6.9
Vermont	6.2	6.9
Virginia	8.6	8.3
Washington	6.3	6.5
West Virginia	9.5	9.7
Wisconsin	7.0	6.9
Wyoming	9.1	8.9
Puerto Rico	12.4	13.0
Virgin Islands	12.3	10.4
Guam	- - -	7.9
American Samoa	3.3	2.8
Northern Marianas	7.0	8.5

---Data not available.

[1] Excludes data for the territories.

Note: For information on the relative standard errors of the data and further discussion, see reference 5.

Table 14. Percentage of Live Births By Cesarean Delivery: United States, Each State and Territory, Final 2006 and Preliminary 2007

[By place of residence. Data are based on a continuous file of records received from the states]

Area	2007	2006
United States[1]	31.8	31.1
Alabama	33.8	33.4
Alaska	22.6	23.0
Arizona	26.2	25.6
Arkansas	34.8	33.2

Table 14. (Continued)

Area	2007	2006
California	32.1	31.3
Colorado	25.8	25.3
Connecticut	34.6	34.1
Delaware	32.1	30.7
District of Columbia	32.6	30.6
Florida	37.2	36.1
Georgia	32.0	31.2
Hawaii	26.4	25.6
Idaho	24.0	22.8
Illinois	30.3	29.6
Indiana	29.4	29.0
Iowa	29.4	27.7
Kansas	29.8	29.3
Kentucky	34.6	34.5
Louisiana	35.9	35.5
Maine	30.0	29.9
Maryland	33.1	32.2
Massachusetts	33.5	33.2
Michigan	30.4	29.8
Minnesota	26.2	25.4
Mississippi	36.2	35.4
Missouri	30.3	30.2
Montana	29.4	28.0
Nebraska	30.9	28.8
Nevada	33.1	32.2
New Hampshire	30.8	29.9
New Jersey	38.3	37.4
New Mexico	23.3	23.3
New York	33.7	32.6
North Carolina	30.7	29.9
North Dakota	28.4	27.8
Ohio	29.8	29.3
Oklahoma	33.6	33.3
Oregon	28.2	28.2
Pennsylvania	30.1	29.7

Table 14. (Continued)

Area	2007	2006
Rhode Island	32.2	31.1
South Carolina	33.4	32.9
South Dakota	26.6	27.0
Tennessee	33.3	32.4
Texas	33.7	33.2
Utah	22.2	21.5
Vermont	26.8	26.0
Virginia	33.5	32.4
Washington	29.0	28.4
West Virginia	35.2	35.2
Wisconsin	25.0	24.6
Wyoming	26.9	26.2
Puerto Rico	49.2	48.3
Virgin Islands	- - -	26.3
Guam	26.5	26.7
American Samoa	- - -	- - -
Northern Marianas	17.7	20.3

- - - Data not available.

[1] Excludes data for the territories.

Note: For information on the relative standard errors of the data and further discussion, see reference 5.

Table 15. Percentage of Births Preterm: United States, Each State and Territory, Final 2006 and Preliminary

[By place of residence. Data are based on a continuous file of records received from the states. Preterm is less than 37 completed weeks of gestation]

Area	2007	2006
United States[1]	12.7	12.8
Alabama	16.6	17.1
Alaska	10.4	11.2
Arizona	12.7	13.2
Arkansas	13.9	13.7
California	10.9	10.7
Colorado	12.2	12.2
Connecticut	10.5	10.4

Table 15. (Continued)

Area	2007	2006
Delaware	14.3	13.7
District of Columbia	15.6	16.0
Florida	13.8	13.8
Georgia	13.6	14.1
Hawaii	12.4	12.1
Idaho	10.5	11.6
Illinois	13.1	13.3
Indiana	12.9	13.2
Iowa	11.6	11.6
Kansas	11.5	11.8
Kentucky	15.2	15.1
Louisiana	16.5	16.4
Maine	10.6	11.1
Maryland	13.4	13.5
Massachusetts	11.2	11.3
Michigan	12.2	12.5
Minnesota	10.4	10.5
Mississippi	18.3	18.8
Missouri	12.5	12.8
Montana	11.9	11.9
Nebraska	11.9	12.5
Nevada	14.3	14.4
New Hampshire	9.4	10.4
New Jersey	12.7	12.9
New Mexico	12.8	14.1
New York	12.3	12.4
North Carolina	13.3	13.6
North Dakota	11.6	12.1
Ohio	13.2	13.3
Oklahoma	13.5	13.9
Oregon	10.3	10.3
Pennsylvania	11.8	11.8
Rhode Island	12.0	12.6
South Carolina	15.5	15.4
South Dakota	12.6	12.7

Table 15. (Continued)

Area	2007	2006
Tennessee	14.2	14.8
Texas	13.6	13.7
Utah	10.9	11.5
Vermont	9.2	9.6
Virginia	12.1	12.0
Washington	10.6	11.0
West Virginia	13.9	14.0
Wisconsin	11.1	11.4
Wyoming	12.7	12.8
Puerto Rico	19.4	19.9
Virgin Islands	14.8	15.6
Guam	- - -	17.7
American Samoa	- - -	- - -
Northern Marianas	11.3	15.9

- - - Data not available.

[1] Excludes data for the territories.

Note: For information on the relative standard errors of the data and further discussion, see reference 5.

- The preliminary **rate of low birthweight** (LBW, less than 2,500 grams) also declined slightly in 2007, to 8.2 percent from 8.3 percent in 2006 (Table 8). The percentage of infants born at LBW had been rising fairly steadily since the mid-1980s (6.7 percent in 1984) (1). The rate of very low birthweight (less than 1,500 grams) was unchanged at 1.5 percent, but the percentage of moderately low birthweight infants declined from 6.8 to 6.7 between 2006 and 2007 (data not shown). Small declines in total LBW were reported for each of the largest racial and Hispanic origin groups: non- Hispanic white (7.3 to 7.2 percent), non-Hispanic black (14.0 to 13.8 percent), and Hispanic infants (7.0 to 6.9 percent).

REFERENCES

[1] Martin JA; Hamilton BE; Sutton PD. et al. Births: Final data for 2006. *National vital statistics reports; vol 57* no 7. Hyattsville, MD: National Center for Health Statistics. 2009. Available from: http://www.cdc.gov /nchs/data/nvsr/nvsr57/nvsr57_07.pdf.

[2]   Hamilton BE; Martin JA; Ventura SJ. Births: Preliminary data for 2006.*National vital statistics reports; vol 56* no 7. Hyattsville, MD: National Center for Health Statistics. 2007. Available from: http://www.cdc.gov/nchs/data/nvsr/nvsr56/nvsr56_07.pdf.

[3]   National Center for Health Statistics. Vital statistics of theUnited States, 2003, volume I, natality. Available from: http://www.cdc.gov/nchs/datawh/statab/unpubd/natality/natab2003.htm.

[4]   Ventura SJ; Bachrach CA. Nonmarital childbearing in theUnited States, 1940–99. *National vital statistics reports; vol 48* no 16. Hyattsville, MD: National Center for Health Statistics. 2000. Available from: http://www.cdc.gov/nchs/data/nvsr/nvsr48/nvs48_16.pdf.

[5]   Hamilton BE; Martin JA; Ventura SJ. Births: Preliminary data for 2005.*National vital statistics reports; vol 55* no 11. Hyattsville, MD: National Center for Health Statistics. 2006. Available from: http://www.cdc.gov/nchs/data/nvsr/nvsr55/nvsr55_11.pdf.

[6]   National Center for Health Statistics. Detailed technical notes—2006—natality. Available from: http://www.cdc.gov/nchs/births.htm.

[7]   National Center for Health Statistics. U.S. Certificate of Live Birth.2003. Available from: http://www.cdc.gov/nchs/data/dvs/birth11-03 final-acc.pdf.

[8]   National Center for Health Statistics. 2003 revision of the U.S.Standard Certificate of Live Birth. 2003. Available from: http://www.cdc.gov/nchs/vital_certs_rev.htm.

[9]   National Center for Health Statistics. Report of the Panel to Evaluate the U.S. Standard Certificates and Reports. 2000. Available from: http://www.cdc.gov/nchs/data/dvs/panelreport_acc.pdf.

[10]   Office of Management and Budget. Revisions to the standards for the classification of federal data on race and ethnicity. Federal Register 62FR58781–58790. October 30, 1997. Available from: http://www.whitehouse.gov/omb/fedreg/ombdir15.html.

[11]   Office of Management and Budget. Race and ethnic standards for federal statistics and administrative reporting. Statistical Policy Directive 15. May 12, 1977.

[12]   Ingram DD; Parker JD; Schenker N. et al. United States Census 2000 with bridged race categories. National Center for Health Statistics. Vital Health Stat 2 (135). 2003. Available from: http://www.cdc.gov/nchs/data/series/sr_02/sr02_135.pdf.

[13]   Johnson D. Coding and editing multiple race. Presented at the 2004 Joint Meeting of NAPHSIS and VSCP. Portland, Oregon. June 6–10, 2004. Available from: http://www.naphsis.org/index.asp?downloadid=75.

[14] Weed JA; Coding and editing multiple race. Presented at the 2004 Joint Meeting of NAPHSIS and VSCP. Portland, Oregon. June 6–10, 2004. Available from: http://www.cdc.gov/nchs/data/dvs/multiple_race_docu_5-10-04.pdf.

[15] Hamilton BE; Ventura SJ. Characteristics of births to single- and multiple-race women: California, Hawaii, Pennsylvania, Utah, and Washington, 2003. *National vital statistics reports; vol 55* no 15. Hyattsville, MD: National Center for Health Statistics. 2007. Available from: http://www.cdc.gov/nchs/data/nvsr/nvsr55/nvsr55_15.pdf.

[16] National Center for Health Statistics. Postcensal estimates of the resident population of the United States as of July 1, 2007, by year, state and county, age, bridged race, sex, and Hispanic origin (vintage 2007). File pcen _v2007_y07.txt (ASCII). Released September 5, 2008. Available from: http://www.cdc.gov/nchs/about/major/dvs/popbridge/datadoc.htm.

[17] U.S. Census Bureau. America's families and living arrangements: 2007. Fertility and Family Statistics Branch. Available from: http://www. census.gov/population/www/socdemo/hh-fam.html.

TECHNICAL NOTES

Nature and Sources of Data

Preliminary data for 2007 are based on a substantial proportion of births for that year (98.7 percent, see Table 10). For 47 of the 50 states and the District of Columbia, over 99 percent of births are included; for Louisiana, over 90 percent are included. The percent completeness for two states, Georgia and Michigan, was lower, at 86.4 and 80.2, respectively, but considered complete enough to provide reliable state-specific estimates. For information and further discussion on the criteria of reliable estimates, see Births: Preliminary Data for 2005 (5). The data for 2007 are based on a continuous receipt and processing of statistical records through July 17, 2008, by the Centers for Disease Control and Prevention's (CDC) National Center for Health Statistics (NCHS). NCHS receives the data from the states' vital registration systems through the Vital Statistics Cooperative Program. In this report, U.S. totals include only events occurring within the 50 states and the District of Columbia. Data for Puerto Rico, the Virgin Islands, American Samoa, and Northern Marianas are included in tables showing data by state, but are not included in U.S. totals (see Tables 6 and 11–15). Data for Guam were not available as of release of the 2007 preliminary file and are not included in this report. Detailed information on reporting completeness and imputation procedures may be found in the "Detailed technical notes— 2006—natality" (6).

To produce the preliminary estimates shown in this report, records in the file were weighted using independent control counts of all 2007 births by state of occurrence. Detailed information on weighting and the reliability of estimates also may be found elsewhere (5).

1989 and 2003 U.S. Standard Certificates of Live Birth

This report includes selected 2006 data on items which are collected on *both* the 1989 Revision of the U.S. Standard Certificate of Live Birth (unrevised) and 2003 Revision of the U.S. Standard Certificate of Live Birth (revised). The 2003 revision is described in detail elsewhere (1, 7–9). Twenty-two states (California, Colorado, Delaware, Florida, Idaho, Indiana, Iowa, Kansas, Kentucky, Nebraska, New Hampshire, New York state (excluding New York City), North Dakota, Ohio, Pennsylvania, South Carolina, South Dakota, Tennessee, Texas, Vermont, Washington, and Wyoming) and Puerto Rico implemented the revised birth certificate as of January 1, 2007. Two additional states, Georgia and Michigan, implemented the revised birth certificate in 2007, but after January 1 for Georgia, and for most, but not all, facilities for Michigan. These 24 revised states represent 60 percent of all births in 2007.

Data items exclusive to either the 1989 or the 2003 birth certificate revision are not shown in this report. A forthcoming report will present selected data exclusive to the 2003 revision from the final data file for 2007.

Hispanic Origin and Race

Hispanic Origin

Hispanic origin and race are reported separately on the birth certificate. Data shown by race (i.e., AIAN and API) include persons of Hispanic or non-Hispanic origin, and data for Hispanic origin include all persons of Hispanic origin of any race. Data for non- Hispanic persons are shown separately according to the race of the mother because there are substantial differences in fertility and maternal and infant health characteristics between Hispanic and non-Hispanic white women. Items asking for the Hispanic origin of the mother have been included on the birth certificates of all states and the District of Columbia, the Virgin Islands, and

Guam since 1993, and on the birth certificate of Puerto Rico starting in 2005 (1). American Samoa and Northern Marianas do not collect this information.

Single, Multiple, and 'Bridged' Race

The 2003 revision of the U.S. Standard Certificate of Live Birth allows the reporting of more than one race (multiple races) for each parent (7) in accordance with the revised standards issued by the Office of Management and Budget (OMB) in 1997 (10,11). Information on this change is presented in several recent reports (1,11,12).

In 2007, 27 states reported multiple-race data: California, Colorado, Delaware, Florida, Georgia (for births occurring after January 1 only), Idaho, Indiana, Iowa, Kansas, Kentucky, Michigan (for births at most facilities), Nebraska, New Hampshire, New York state (excluding New York City), North Dakota, Ohio, Pennsylvania, South Carolina, South Dakota, Tennessee, Texas, Vermont, Washington, and Wyoming, which used the 2003 revision of the U.S. Standard Certificate of Live Birth, as well as Hawaii, Minnesota, and Utah, which used the 1989 revision of the U.S. Standard Certificate of Live Birth. Puerto Rico, which revised its birth certificate in 2005, reported race according to the 1989 revision of the U.S. Standard Certificate of Live Birth. The 27 states accounted for 63 percent of births in the United States in 2007. Data from the vital records of the remaining 23 states, New York City, and the District of Columbia are based on the 1989 revision of the U.S. Standard Certificate of Live Birth that follows the 1977 OMB standard, allowing only a single race to be reported (10–12).

To provide uniformity and comparability of the data during the transition period, before all or most of the data are available in the new multiple-race format, it was necessary to "bridge" the responses of those who reported more than one race (multiple race) to a single race. The bridging procedure for multiple-race mothers and fathers is based on the procedure used to bridge the multiple-race population estimates (see "Population denominators") (13,14). Information detailing the processing and tabulation of data by race is presented elsewhere (1). A recent report describes multiple-race birth data for 2003 (15).

Change in Imputation of Race for Hispanic Women

Starting with the 2006 data year for data on the revised birth certificate, the race edit was modified slightly to take into account differences in the race distribution for births to Hispanic women compared with all births. A recent report provided more detailed information about the modification to the race edit and its impact (1).

Marital Status

National estimates of births to unmarried women are based on two methods of determining marital status. For 2006 and 2007, birth certificates in 48 states and the District of Columbia included a direct question about the mother's marital status; in two of these states, California and Nevada, a direct question is part of the electronic birth registration process but does not appear on certified or paper copies of the birth certificate. The question in most states is: "Mother married? (At birth, conception, or any time between) (Yes or no)." Marital status is inferred in Michigan and New York. A birth is inferred as nonmarital if a paternity acknowledgment was filed or if the father's name is missing from the birth certificate (listed in respective priority-of-use order).

Population Denominators

Birth and fertility rates for 2007 shown in this report are based on population estimates based on the 2000 census, as of July 1, 2007. These population estimates are available on the NCHS website (16). The production of these population estimates is described in detail in a recent report (1).

Information on the national estimates of births to unmarried women (i.e., methods of determining marital status) and the computation of preliminary birth rates for unmarried women is presented elsewhere (2,5). The birth rate for unmarried women for 2007 is estimated on the basis of population distributions by marital status provided by the U.S. Census Bureau as of March 2007 applied to the national population estimates as of July 1, 2007 (4,16,17). Both population files are based on the 2000 census.

The nonmarital birth rate shown in the preliminary report thus differs from those published by NCHS in the annual final reports, which are based on populations estimated from 3-year averages of the marital status distributions rather than a single year, as shown here (4). Population estimates for a single year are not an adequate basis for computing age-specific birth rates for unmarried women—these rates are available only in reports based on final data.

The populations used in this report were produced under a collaborative arrangement with the U.S. Census Bureau and are based on the 2000 census counts. Reflecting the new guidelines issued in 1997 by OMB, the 2000 census included an option for persons to report more than one race as appropriate for themselves and household members (10). In order to produce birth and fertility rates by race, bridging the reported population data for multiple-race persons back to single-race categories was necessary. For detailed information on the revised OMB standards on race reporting and procedures used to produce the "bridged" populations, see "United States Census 2000 with Bridged Race Categories" (12).

Computing Rates and Percentages; Reliability of Estimates

For information and further discussion on computing rates and percentages and the relative standard errors of the data, see Births: Preliminary Data for 2005 (5).

ACKNOWLEDGMENTS

This report was prepared under the general direction of Charles J. Rothwell, Director of the Division of Vital Statistics (DVS) and Stephanie J. Ventura, Chief of the Reproductive Statistics Branch (RSB). Nicholas F. Pace, Chief of the Systems, Programming, and Statistical Resources Branch (SPSRB), and Steve Steimel, Candace Cosgrove, Annie Liu, Jordan Sacks, Manju Sharma, and Bonita Gross provided computer programming support and statistical tables. Yashodhara Patel of RSB also provided statistical tables. Steve Steimel and Candace Cosgrove of SPSRB prepared the natality file. Michelle J.K. Osterman of RSB provided content review. Staff of the Data Acquisition and Evaluation Branch carried out quality evaluation and acceptance procedures for the state data files on which this report is based. The Registration Methods staff of DVS consulted with state vital statistics offices regarding the collection of birth certificate data. This report was edited by Jane Sudol and Demarius V. Miller, CDC/CCHIS/NCHM/Division of Creative Services, Writer- Editor Services Branch, and typeset by Jacqueline M. Davis of CDC/CCHIS/NCHM/Division of Creative Services. Graphics were produced by Sarah Hinkle, CDC/CCHIS/NCHM/Division of Creative Services.

INDEX

A

abortion, viii, ix, x, 2, 19, 29, 55, 68, 78, 82, 83, 85, 87, 88, 89, 92, 94

abstinence, viii, 34, 35, 36, 37, 38, 45, 48, 50, 51, 61, 62, 65, 67, 68, 69, 70, 71, 72, 73, 74, 75, 79

abusive, 30, 41

ACF, 43, 44

achievement, 40

administration, 81, 82

administrative, 20, 21, 134

adolescent female, 20

adolescents, 7, 27, 32, 35, 36, 45, 50, 51, 69, 72, 73, 79, 80, 90

adult, viii, 2, 3, 22, 25, 47, 49

adulthood, 3, 58

adults, vii, 1, 3, 5, 26, 28, 30, 31, 32, 34, 39, 48, 51, 72

advertising, 40

affiliates, 80, 86

African American, 5, 17

African Americans, 17

after-school, 47

aging, 6, 32

Alabama, 102, 116, 122, 124, 126, 128, 129, 131

Alaska, 10, 33, 55, 72, 101, 105, 107, 109, 110, 112, 115, 116, 117, 118, 119, 121, 122, 124, 126, 128, 129, 131

Alaska Natives, 10, 33, 55

Alaskan Native, 10, 56

alcohol, 28, 45, 72

alternative, 17, 35, 46, 69, 71

ambiguity, 17

amendments, 94

American Civil Liberties Union, 95

American Community Survey, 56

American Indian, 5, 10, 15, 33, 55, 56, 101, 105, 107, 109, 110, 112, 115, 116, 117, 118, 119, 121

American Indians, 10, 33, 55

analysts, viii, 2, 3, 5, 17, 22, 23, 38, 42, 44, 49, 57, 58, 65

API, 99, 100, 101, 102, 136

application, 57

appropriations, ix, 36, 68, 70, 77, 78, 80, 82, 84, 86, 88, 93, 94, 95

appropriations bills, ix, 77, 80

Appropriations Committee, 80, 82, 84, 93, 95

argument, 26, 94, 95

Arizona, 102, 117, 122, 124, 126, 128, 129, 131

Arkansas, 117, 122, 124, 126, 128, 129, 131

Asian, 5, 10, 11, 15, 33, 55, 56, 99, 105, 107, 109, 110, 112, 115, 116, 117, 118, 119, 121

Atlantic, 56, 58, 60, 64

attitudes, viii, 2, 3, 26, 29, 72

authority, 80, 81, 82, 90

avoidance, 72

awareness, ix, 78, 82

B

babies, 7, 11, 13, 17, 40, 61

baby boom, 24, 99, 101

barriers, 42, 89

behavior, 39, 40, 46, 49, 72

behavioral problems, 5, 30

benefits, 21, 32, 43, 47, 57, 63

biological parents, vii, 1, 3, 4, 5, 27, 30, 48, 49, 50, 54

birth control, 35, 39, 74

birth rate, x, 6, 7, 8, 10, 13, 23, 24, 32, 33, 55, 61, 68, 98, 100, 101, 102, 103, 104, 105, 108, 116, 120, 138

birthweight, 121, 128, 133

black women, 5, 9, 10, 17, 26, 33, 55, 61, 100

Blacks, 57

block grants, 75

boys, 62

brothers, 50

Bush Administration, 38, 42, 50

C

campaigns, 40, 42, 72

career counseling, 38

career development, 79

causal relationship, 18

CDC, 62, 93, 99, 104, 135, 139

Census Bureau, 6, 23, 25, 54, 55, 56, 57, 58, 59, 60, 61, 135, 138

Centers for Disease Control, 57, 58, 62, 75, 79, 93, 98, 135

certificate, 136, 137, 138, 139

cervical cancer, 45, 79

child abuse, 81, 82

child development, 35, 69

child poverty, 32

Child Support Enforcement, 21, 34, 44, 46, 58, 64

child welfare, 32

child well-being, 30

childbearing, vii, viii, x, 1, 2, 4, 11, 13, 17, 18, 22, 23, 26, 31, 32, 34, 39, 40, 46, 47, 49, 58, 60, 64, 98, 103, 134

childhood, 30

childrearing, 22, 64

classes, 39, 46, 72

classification, 134

clients, 63, 79, 80, 81, 85, 89, 94

clinics, 79, 80, 84, 89

coercion, 45, 79, 81, 82

Colorado, 44, 102, 117, 122, 124, 126, 128, 130, 131, 136, 137

Columbia, 64, 94, 102, 103, 117, 122, 124, 126, 128, 130, 132, 135, 136, 137, 138

Committee on Appropriations, 84, 94, 95

communication, 34, 38, 43

communication skills, 34, 38, 43

communities, 41, 43

community, viii, 21, 28, 38, 41, 42, 43, 47, 61, 62, 67, 69, 75, 80, 92

competition, 26, 81

compilation, 74

complexity, 6, 23

compliance, 44, 88

components, 34, 38, 39, 44, 62

computing, 138, 139

conception, 22, 138

condom, 58, 79

conflict, 40, 42, 48, 89, 94

conflict resolution, 40, 42

congress, 84, 94

Congress, 2, 4, 42, 43, 47, 49, 50, 51, 54, 62, 63, 64, 67, 68, 77, 78, 86, 87, 94, 95

Connecticut, 72, 117, 122, 124, 126, 128, 130, 131
consensus, 13, 50
Consolidated Appropriations Act, 81, 82, 84, 93, 94
contraceptives, 20, 37, 39, 58, 74, 90
contracts, 43, 70, 90, 91
control, vii, viii, x, 2, 19, 36, 38, 39, 41, 50, 95, 97, 136
control group, 36, 38, 41, 50
costs, 4, 5, 19, 31, 32, 60, 61, 81
counseling, x, 37, 38, 43, 45, 75, 78, 79, 81, 82, 83, 88, 89
couples, viii, 2, 16, 17, 22, 24, 27, 40, 41, 49, 56, 63, 64, 65
Court of Appeals, 94
credit, 63
criminal justice, 31
crisis intervention, 38
CRS, 2, 61, 62, 63, 68, 77, 85, 90, 94
culture, 38
Current Population Survey, 56, 60

D

Dallas, 41
death, 87
decisions, 37, 73, 74
Deficit Reduction Act, 40, 42, 47, 62, 63
definition, 70, 89
delinquent behavior, 46
delivery, x, 35, 44, 47, 69, 70, 79, 81, 83, 97, 98, 104, 106, 121
demographic characteristics, 9
demographic factors, 18, 22, 24, 31, 54
Department of Health and Human Services, ix, 7, 8, 9, 12, 14, 35, 43, 54, 56, 57, 58, 61, 62, 63, 64, 68, 69, 77, 78, 84, 88, 92, 93, 95, 97
dignity, 46, 79
directives, 37
discrimination, 82, 88, 89

distribution, 14, 81, 92, 137
District of Columbia, 94, 102, 103, 122, 124, 126, 128, 130, 132, 135, 136, 137, 138
District of Columbia Circuit, 94
divorce, 27, 28, 31
doctors, 21
domestic violence, 40, 41
drinking, 39
drug use, 72
drugs, 28, 39
duration, 4, 16, 27, 28

E

earnings, 32, 43, 44
economic stability, 43
economic status, 21, 41
economically disadvantaged, 6
educated women, 9, 14
education, v, viii, ix, 35, 36, 37, 38, 61, 62, 67, 68, 71, 73, 74, 75, 77, 80, 82, 84, 85, 86, 87, 93, 94, 95
educational background, 11
emotional, 3, 5, 19, 21, 25, 30, 35, 42, 49, 74
emotional health, 35, 74
employment, 26, 43, 44
empowered, 35, 74
England, 54, 56, 59
enrollment, 36
environment, 48
equity, 21
ethnic groups, 9, 26, 33
ethnicity, viii, 2, 9, 10, 19, 55, 134
expenditures, 31, 62, 73
experimental design, 41

F

faith, 38
family, ix, 3, 5, 6, 16, 21, 26, 27, 28, 31, 34, 35, 39, 41, 45, 46, 48, 49, 50, 55, 69, 70,

73, 75, 77, 78, 79, 81, 82, 83, 85, 87, 90, 91, 92, 93, 94, 95, 102
family life, 3, 49
family members, 28
family planning, ix, 34, 45, 48, 73, 75, 77, 78, 79, 81, 82, 83, 85, 87, 90, 91, 92, 94, 95
family structure, 48, 55
fatherhood, 4, 20, 34, 40, 42, 43, 44, 45, 47, 48, 50, 63, 65
February, 42, 47, 55, 57, 58, 59, 61, 62, 63, 64, 81, 95
federal funds, ix, 36, 71, 78, 83, 85, 86
federal government, viii, ix, 1, 19, 31, 34, 36, 38, 42, 49, 77, 85
Federal Register, ix, 78, 82, 88, 94, 95, 96, 134
fee, 45, 57, 79
females, 5, 11, 13, 20, 24, 29, 34, 37, 54, 55, 68, 100
fertility, viii, x, 2, 3, 6, 19, 32, 33, 40, 49, 57, 71, 98, 99, 100, 102, 103, 105, 108, 116, 136, 138
fertility rate, x, 32, 33, 98, 99, 100, 102, 103, 105, 108, 116, 138
fertilization, 27
financial support, 21, 46
first-time, 11
fluctuations, 7, 8
fragmentation, 31
freedom, 25, 30
fulfillment, 22
funding, viii, ix, 35, 36, 37, 38, 42, 43, 47, 48, 50, 51, 61, 65, 67, 68, 70, 71, 72, 73, 75, 77, 78, 79, 80, 81, 84, 85, 94
funds, ix, 13, 36, 37, 40, 43, 47, 49, 61, 62, 68, 71, 75, 78, 79, 80, 81, 82, 83, 85, 86, 87, 88, 92

G

General Accounting Office, 62, 86, 95
generation, 24, 33, 102

Georgia, 60, 102, 117, 122, 124, 126, 128, 130, 132, 135, 136, 137
Germany, 57
gestation, x, 98, 104, 120, 121, 122, 131
girls, 18, 29, 37, 39, 62
goals, 21, 40, 44, 47, 48, 72
government, iv, viii, ix, 1, 14, 19, 31, 34, 36, 38, 40, 42, 49, 62, 77, 82, 85, 91
Government Accountability Office, 63, 86
GPO, 95
grades, viii, 67
grants, ix, 35, 40, 42, 44, 45, 47, 63, 69, 70, 75, 77, 78, 79, 80, 88, 90, 91
groups, viii, x, 2, 4, 6, 9, 13, 26, 33, 34, 38, 43, 49, 50, 55, 62, 65, 98, 100, 101, 102, 103, 105, 106, 133
growth, 6, 25, 32, 61, 91, 92
Guam, 119, 124, 126, 127, 129, 131, 133, 135, 137
guidelines, 44, 138

H

Harvard, 54, 60
Hawaii, 103, 117, 122, 124, 126, 128, 130, 132, 135, 137
Head Start, 57
health, ix, 21, 32, 35, 36, 37, 38, 42, 45, 69, 71, 77, 78, 79, 80, 82, 86, 88, 89, 90, 98, 136
health care, ix, 32, 38, 42, 78, 80, 82, 88, 89
health care professionals, 88
health care system, 42
health problems, 71
health services, ix, 45, 77, 79
healthcare, 93
HHS, ix, 35, 37, 40, 41, 43, 45, 54, 58, 61, 63, 68, 69, 72, 75, 77, 78, 80, 82, 84, 88, 89, 92, 93, 95
high school, 32, 37, 39, 40, 42, 44, 47, 62
Hispanic origin, x, 55, 97, 98, 99, 100, 101, 102, 103, 105, 106, 107, 108, 109, 110,

111, 112, 113, 114, 115, 116, 119, 121, 133, 135, 136
Hispanic population, 6, 33
Hispanics, 6, 10, 18, 33, 57
HIV, 35, 45, 51, 74, 79, 93
HIV/AIDS, 35, 74, 79
hospitals, 70, 80, 87
House, 63, 64, 84, 86, 87, 88, 94
House Ways and Means Subcommittee, 63
household, 3, 4, 56, 60, 138
households, 16, 27, 49, 63, 70
housing, 61, 69
human, 71
husband, 3, 20, 48, 60

infections, 62
infertility, 45, 79, 90
inheritance, 21
initiation, 39
innocence, 72
Inspector General, 94
institutions, ix, 78, 88
insurance, 21
integration, 79
interaction, 70
interference, 14
interstate, 47
intervention, 38, 39, 46
intimacy, 25

I

Idaho, 103, 117, 122, 124, 126, 128, 130, 132, 136, 137
identification, 36
identity, 21, 25
Illinois, 103, 117, 122, 124, 126, 128, 130, 132
immigration, 33
impact analysis, 50
implants, 58
implementation, 45, 65, 88, 91
incarceration, 19, 32
incentives, 40, 45
incest, 81, 82, 87
incidence, 20, 22
income, vii, viii, 1, 2, 3, 5, 9, 16, 19, 30, 34, 41, 42, 44, 45, 47, 54, 60, 63, 72, 79, 80, 91
income support, viii, 2, 34
income tax, 63
incomes, 30, 80
independence, 27, 39
Indian, 40, 43
Indiana, 102, 103, 117, 122, 124, 126, 128, 130, 132, 136, 137
Indians, 6, 33
infant care, 83
infants, x, 46, 57, 98, 101, 120, 133

J

job preparation, 40
job training, 43, 69
jobs, 11, 26, 34, 44, 65, 89
Jordan, 139
justice, 31

K

Kentucky, 102, 103, 117, 123, 125, 126, 128, 130, 132, 136, 137

L

labor force, 22, 26
language, 48, 81, 82
law, ix, 36, 37, 40, 47, 62, 71, 78, 81, 82, 83, 84, 89
laws, 47, 81, 82, 88
legislation, viii, 50, 67
lifestyle, 34
lifetime, 26, 32
living arrangements, 50, 59, 135
living environment, 49
local government, 38, 42, 82

logistics, 93
loneliness, 39
Louisiana, 102, 103, 117, 123, 125, 126, 128, 130, 132, 135
love, 39, 48
low birthweight, x, 97, 98, 99, 121, 133
lower-income, 45, 79
low-income, 41, 42, 44, 45, 47, 72, 79, 80, 91

M

Madison, 56
Maine, 72, 117, 123, 125, 126, 128, 130, 132
maintenance, 40, 48, 62
males, 10, 24, 55, 79
maltreatment, 28
management, 39
manpower, 79
marital status, x, 21, 54, 65, 97, 138
marriages, 16, 22, 26, 28, 40, 46, 60
married couples, viii, 2, 22, 27, 40, 50, 63
married women, 16, 22, 24
Maryland, 44, 103, 117, 123, 125, 127, 128, 130, 132
Massachusetts, 44, 117, 123, 125, 127, 128, 130, 132
matching funds, 61, 75
maternal, 48, 98, 136
measures, x, 6, 17, 36, 47, 49, 98, 103
media, 42, 43, 72, 95
median, viii, 2, 22, 24, 27, 28, 74
mediation, 42, 43, 44
Medicaid, 37, 57, 73
medical care, 81
medical services, 45, 75
men, viii, 2, 11, 16, 19, 20, 24, 26, 28, 32, 42, 44, 47, 50, 55
mentoring, 38, 39, 43
messages, 37, 74
Mexico, 103, 118, 123, 125, 127, 128, 130, 132
middle-aged, 65

Minnesota, 72, 103, 118, 123, 125, 127, 128, 130, 132, 137
minorities, 6, 33
minority, 6, 10, 18, 33
minority groups, 6, 33
minors, 81
miscarriage, 55
misleading, 28, 75
Mississippi, 103, 118, 123, 125, 127, 128, 130, 132
Missouri, 41, 44, 103, 118, 123, 125, 127, 128, 130, 132
MOE, 62
money, 65
Montana, 72, 118, 123, 125, 127, 128, 130, 132
motherhood, 9, 14, 34
mothers, vii, viii, 2, 3, 4, 6, 9, 10, 11, 13, 14, 16, 17, 18, 19, 21, 32, 34, 41, 42, 46, 48, 54, 56, 60, 64, 103, 120, 137

N

nation, vii, viii, 2, 4, 6, 19, 25, 32, 33, 49, 51
Native Hawaiian, 33, 55
natural, 25, 33, 45, 79, 90
NC, 93
Nebraska, 118, 123, 125, 127, 128, 130, 132, 136, 137
negative consequences, 13, 61, 68, 75
negative outcomes, 4, 49
Nevada, 103, 118, 123, 125, 127, 128, 130, 132, 138
New Jersey, 72, 102, 103, 118, 123, 125, 127, 128, 130, 132
New Mexico, 103, 118, 123, 125, 127, 128, 130, 132
New York, iii, iv, 55, 60, 63, 102, 103, 118, 123, 125, 127, 128, 130, 132, 136, 137, 138
New York Times, 60
noncustodial fathers, 19, 42, 43, 44
non-profit, 45

North Carolina, 103, 118, 123, 125, 127, 128, 130, 132
nurses, 39

O

obligation, 25, 89, 91
obligations, 42, 47
Office of Management and Budget, 108, 116, 119, 121, 134, 137
Ohio, 41, 102, 103, 118, 123, 125, 127, 129, 130, 132, 136, 137
Oklahoma, 103, 118, 123, 125, 127, 129, 130, 132
old-fashioned, 48
OMB, 105, 108, 110, 113, 116, 119, 121, 137, 138
opposition, 81
oral, 58, 62, 75
Oregon, 118, 123, 125, 127, 129, 130, 132, 134, 135

P

Pacific Islander, 10, 15, 33, 55, 56, 99, 105, 107, 109, 110, 112, 115, 116, 117, 118, 119, 121
Pacific Islanders, 10
pap smear, 75
parent involvement, 43
parental participation, 93
parenthood, 25, 50
parenting, 22, 35, 39, 42, 43, 68, 69, 70
parents, vii, 1, 3, 4, 5, 16, 17, 21, 22, 27, 28, 30, 32, 35, 41, 42, 43, 44, 46, 47, 48, 49, 50, 54, 58, 59, 60, 65, 69, 70, 71, 72
partnerships, 69
paternity, 18, 19, 20, 21, 47, 138
patients, x, 78, 88, 89
peer, 37, 38, 42, 43, 74, 75
peer support, 37, 42, 43
penalties, 47

penalty, 63
Pennsylvania, 72, 102, 103, 118, 123, 125, 127, 129, 130, 132, 135, 136, 137
perception, 5, 13, 16, 59
periodic, 83
permit, 50
personal responsibility, 42
PHS, 54, 62
physical abuse, 28
physicians, 88
planning, ix, 34, 45, 48, 51, 69, 73, 75, 77, 78, 79, 80, 81, 82, 83, 85, 87, 90, 91, 92, 94, 95
policymakers, 4, 13, 25, 41, 48, 51
poor, 30, 50
population, 4, 6, 10, 23, 24, 28, 29, 31, 32, 33, 40, 44, 55, 59, 61, 91, 92, 100, 102, 103, 105, 116, 135, 137, 138
population group, 4, 103
population growth, 6, 32, 91, 92
postponement, viii, 2, 11, 22, 24, 58
postsecondary education, 26
poverty, 5, 16, 30, 31, 32, 46, 54, 60, 80
power, 20
pre-existing, 94
pregnancy, viii, 2, 4, 11, 22, 28, 32, 34, 35, 36, 37, 38, 39, 46, 47, 51, 55, 56, 58, 59, 61, 62, 64, 67, 68, 69, 70, 71, 72, 74, 75, 81, 82, 83, 85
pregnant, viii, x, 11, 20, 27, 35, 55, 67, 68, 69, 71, 78, 82, 83, 85, 88
pregnant women, x, 78, 82, 83, 88
prenatal care, 83
President Bush, ix, 73, 78, 80, 81, 84
pressure, 22, 37, 38, 74, 75
prevention, viii, 2, 4, 34, 35, 37, 38, 45, 51, 56, 62, 67, 68, 69, 70, 72, 74, 79
preventive, ix, 77, 79
privacy, 46, 79
private, 35, 38, 40, 42, 43, 45, 48, 49, 61, 69, 75, 90, 91
probability, 39
problem-solving, 42
problem-solving skills, 42

production, 138
profit, 45
programming, 139
protection, 37, 74, 89
psychosocial factors, 93
public finance, 50
public funds, 13
public health, 70
Public Health Service, 35, 45, 63, 67, 69, 77,
    88, 90, 95
public policy, vii, viii, 2, 4, 21, 34
public schools, 70
public service, 61, 75
public support, 62, 81
Puerto Rico, 102, 103, 119, 124, 126, 127,
    129, 131, 133, 135, 136, 137

R

race categories, 108, 116, 119, 121, 134, 139
racial differences, 18
random assignment, 38, 41
range, 34, 40, 47, 90
rape, 81, 82, 87
reality, 16, 51
recognition, viii, 1, 34, 67
recovery, 46
regression, 31
regulation, 82, 83, 89
regulations, 80, 82, 83, 89, 91, 92, 94, 95
regulatory requirements, 83
relationship, 9, 16, 17, 18, 21, 25, 30, 37, 40,
    41, 71, 74, 93
relationships, 6, 10, 16, 17, 19, 20, 27, 30, 41,
    48, 49, 60, 79
relatives, 60
reliability, 116, 136, 139
religious beliefs, 46, 79, 88, 89
religious groups, 62
replacement rate, 6, 32, 33, 102
resolution, 40, 42, 80, 84
resources, 3, 6, 13, 32, 50, 62, 95

responsiveness, 85
returns, 58
revenue, 32
Rhode Island, 72, 118, 123, 125, 127, 129,
    131, 132
risk, 5, 28, 29, 33, 37, 38, 58, 59
risks, 36, 37, 74
RTI International, 93
rural areas, 79

S

Samoa, 102, 103, 119, 124, 126, 127, 129,
    131, 133, 135, 137
savings, 32, 61
scarce resources, 13
scarcity, 50
SCHIP, 57
school, 5, 30, 32, 36, 37, 39, 40, 42, 44, 46,
    47, 62, 65, 70, 71, 73
scores, 46
security, 21, 46, 48
segmentation, 55
seizure, 47
self-esteem, 21, 59
Senate, 80, 82, 84, 86, 87, 93, 95
separation, 60, 83
sex, viii, 2, 22, 26, 28, 34, 35, 36, 37, 38, 39,
    46, 49, 50, 51, 56, 59, 61, 62, 65, 68, 72,
    73, 74, 75, 135
sexual abuse, 81, 82
sexual activities, 37, 74
sexual activity, viii, 2, 5, 22, 28, 34, 37, 38, 39,
    51, 62, 68, 71, 72, 75, 81, 82, 85
sexual behavior, 28
sexual contact, 20
sexual intercourse, viii, 28, 37, 67, 68, 72
sexuality, 35, 69, 70, 74
sexually transmitted disease, 35, 37, 62, 68,
    74, 79
sexually transmitted diseases, 35, 37, 62, 68,
    74

sexually transmitted infections, 62
sexually-transmitted diseases, 20
shame, 39, 48
shares, 29
shortage, 11, 26
short-term, 40
sibling, 28
sites, 85
skills, 34, 37, 38, 39, 40, 42, 43, 65, 69, 74, 75
social consequences, viii, 1
social policy, 42
social security, 21
Social Security, 44, 46, 47, 57, 71
social services, 35, 68, 69, 75
Social Services, 38
social skills, 40, 69
social welfare, 19
socioeconomic, vii, 1, 3, 30
sociologists, 6, 32
South Carolina, 118, 123, 125, 127, 129, 131, 132, 136, 137
South Dakota, 118, 123, 125, 127, 129, 131, 132, 136, 137
spectrum, 34
sperm, 27, 64
sporadic, 42
sports, 38, 39
spouse, 27, 49
St. Louis, 41
stability, 43, 48, 103
staffing, 61, 75
standard error, 105, 108, 110, 113, 116, 119, 120, 121, 122, 126, 127, 129, 131, 133, 139
standards, 105, 108, 110, 113, 116, 119, 121, 134, 137, 139
State Children's Health Insurance Program, 57
statistics, x, 55, 68, 97, 98, 133, 134, 135, 139
statutes, ix, 78, 83
statutory, 40, 89
statutory provisions, 89
STD, 45, 51, 79
sterilization, 58, 88

stigma, 26, 48
STIs, 62
strategies, 4, 42, 49, 50, 75, 93
strength, 35, 74
stress, 42, 73
students, viii, 36, 37, 62, 67, 70
substance abuse, 28, 41, 45
substitution, 62, 75
supplemental, 79
Supplemental Security Income, 57
survivors, 41
Sweden, 85

T

TANF, 34, 38, 40, 43, 47, 48, 50, 57, 61, 62, 63, 75
taxes, 6, 31, 32
taxpayers, 31, 32
teachers, 72
teaching, 36, 71
technical assistance, 40
teenage girls, viii, 2, 3, 20
teenagers, viii, x, 2, 5, 9, 11, 13, 20, 28, 34, 35, 38, 39, 49, 56, 68, 71, 72, 74, 98, 100, 101, 103
teens, viii, 2, 5, 11, 13, 26, 31, 32, 34, 35, 37, 38, 39, 47, 49, 51, 56, 60, 62, 65, 67, 68, 69, 71, 74, 75, 85
Temporary Assistance for Needy Families, 34, 47, 75
Tennessee, 103, 118, 123, 125, 127, 129, 131, 133, 136, 137
territorial, 80
Texas, 41, 72, 73, 102, 103, 118, 123, 125, 127, 129, 131, 133, 136, 137
third party, 91
training, 42, 43, 69, 79, 88, 91
transition period, 137
transitions, 50
transportation, 45
tribal, 40, 43

trust, 25   vulnerability, 72

U

uniform, 47
uninsured, 80
unions, 11
universe, 10, 26
universities, 70, 80
unmarried men, 26, 28, 47
unmarried women, x, 2, 6, 7, 8, 10, 11, 17, 20,
    22, 23, 24, 29, 30, 33, 46, 48, 55, 61, 98,
    103, 105, 138
upload, 96
Utah, 102, 118, 123, 125, 127, 129, 131, 133,
    135, 137

W

wealth, 41
welfare, viii, 32, 36, 37, 40, 42, 43, 47, 63, 67,
    71
welfare reform, viii, 36, 37, 40, 42, 47, 67, 71
well-being, 3, 25, 30
white women, 10, 17, 18, 33, 99, 102, 136
Wisconsin, 41, 44, 56, 103, 119, 124, 125,
    127, 129, 131, 133
workers, 6, 32
workplace, 65
Wyoming, 72, 119, 124, 126, 127, 129, 131,
    133, 136, 137

V

Vermont, 72, 102, 119, 123, 125, 127, 129,
    131, 133, 136, 137
veterans, 21
violence, 28, 40, 41
violent, 41
visible, 46

Y

young adults, 51
young men, 16
young women, 19, 20, 37